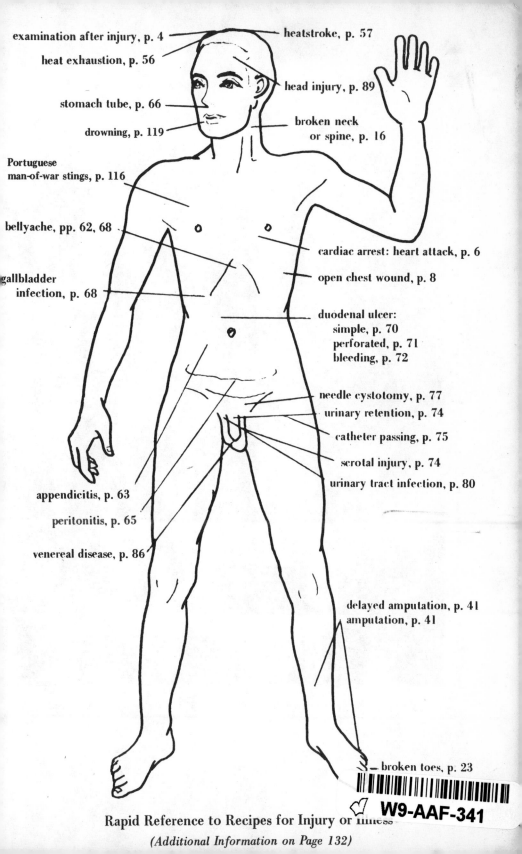

examination after injury, p. 4

heat exhaustion, p. 56

stomach tube, p. 66

drowning, p. 119

Portuguese
man-of-war stings, p. 116

bellyache, pp. 62, 68

gallbladder
infection, p. 68

appendicitis, p. 63

peritonitis, p. 65

venereal disease, p. 86

heatstroke, p. 57

head injury, p. 89

broken neck
or spine, p. 16

cardiac arrest: heart attack, p. 6

open chest wound, p. 8

duodenal ulcer:
simple, p. 70
perforated, p. 71
bleeding, p. 72

needle cystotomy, p. 77
urinary retention, p. 74

catheter passing, p. 75

scrotal injury, p. 74

urinary tract infection, p. 80

delayed amputation, p. 41
amputation, p. 41

broken toes, p. 23

W9-AAF-341

Rapid Reference to Recipes for Injury or Illness

(Additional Information on Page 132)

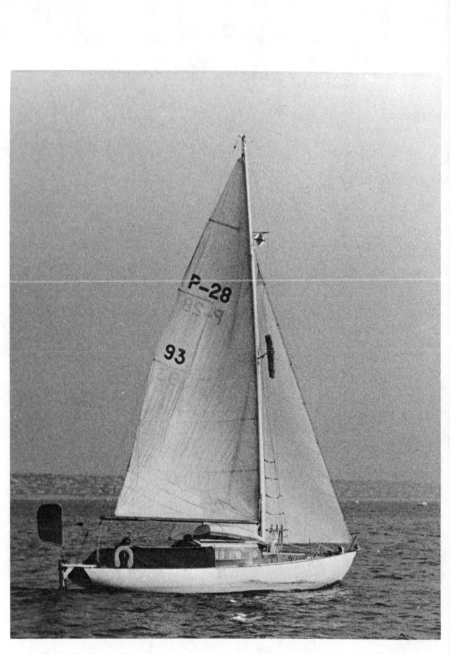

Sloop *Wa* leaving Marina del Rey, Calif., Jan. 3, 1971 for a round-the-world trip.

ADVANCED

First Aid Afloat

by

Peter F. Eastman, M.D.

Second Edition
Revised and Enlarged

Cornell Maritime Press, Inc.

Centreville   Maryland

ISBN 0—87033—169-8

Library of Congress Catalog Card Number: 72-78241

Printed in the United States of America

Copyright © 1972, 1974 by Cornell Maritime Press, Inc.

Fifth Printing, 1979

PREFACE

Advanced First Aid Afloat was born from discussions with son Peter and his wife Addie in May 1970. They were living aboard *Wa*, their 28-foot sloop, in Santa Barbara, California, getting set to sail her around the world. At the time of this writing they have reached Rabaul in the South Pacific.

They cruised to American Samoa in 1968 and were troubled by injury and accident that caused them much unnecessary anxiety for lack of a detailed book on extensive First Aid. They asked me to help avoid this on the proposed trip.

I outlined diagnosis and treatment of common serious injury and illness in ordinary terms. They suggested revisions necessary for clearer understanding and easier use on a boat at sea.

We melded our own and many friends' relevant seafaring experiences to make this more than a dry technical manual.

Lifesaving First Aid demands but three things be done fast. Restore breathing, get the victim out of harm's way, and stop major bleeding. Bleeding is more spectacular but apnea (non-breathing) is a more immediate threat to life and must never be overlooked. Certain situations may change the order of these three actions but all three must always be considered.

When these are controlled, there is time to plan care to sustain the rescued one in good condition until he recovers or gets to a doctor.

Diagnosis and management of fractures—both simple and compound—burns, abdominal pain, genitourinary injuries, severe infections and antibiotic usage, heatstroke and exhaustion, head injury, control of irrational behavior and drugs, wounds and serious dental problems are all discussed.

Drugs and supplies relating to these subjects are presented, as well as a Glossary of medical terms as used.

The Introduction explains briefly how to use this book to best advantage.

Many good men and women, sailors and non-sailors, have bent a hand in this weaving.

Drs. Stanley Christie, Lynn Solomon, Robert Frank and Arthur Sutherland, all from the Palos Verdes Peninsula, California, reinforced my shortage of knowledge in their medical specialties. Alex Okrand, D.D.S., furnished material for the dental section.

Sybil Schwartz, medical librarian, spent many hours digging out reference articles.

Richard Esposito, photographer extraordinary of Balboa Island, California, brought my dreams to pictures before his lens.

My surgical assistants, Duke, Frank, Lou, Mark and Gus, helped immeasurably in our constant search for illustrative material.

My wife, Betty, executed the excellent line drawings.

Finally, Julie Gamble, Debbie Gray and Gretchen Sampson each labored over my almost illegible scrawl and brought it to proper grammatical and beautifully typewritten form.

My heartfelt thanks to all of them. I hope you find their efforts useful.

P.F.E., M.D.

This book is affectionately dedicated to the yacht **Wa,**

PETER, ADDIE AND COCO

CONTENTS

LIST OF ILLUSTRATIONS

Rapid Reference to Recipes for Injury or Illness: Inside back cover
and facing page

INTRODUCTION

Helpful Hints for Use of This Book

Before the start of cruise or race:

1. Master the gist of Chapter I, *First Things First.* If you need this information there will be no time to read up on it.

2. Consult with your physician and druggist concerning purchase of supplies listed in Chapter X.

If disaster strikes:

1. Open the book to the inside front cover. Two human figures surrounded by labels and page numbers provide quick access to cookbook recipes for your needs. These may not be identical with your problem but you will recognize the relevance.

2. When matters are under control after a bit, read on into the discussion sections of each chapter. You will find certain patterns of response common to all stress. The reasons for what you did will become clear. Your judgment grows and anxiety for the continuing care of your patient subsides.

The illustrative cases are true misadventures overcome by courageous sailor men and women. They will give you a better idea of how things may actually look if someone is injured or becomes seriously ill.

Chapter I
FIRST THINGS FIRST

Your cruising ketch is four days out of Los Angeles Harbor toward Diamond Head. At 0700 hours a sleepy helmsman invites an unintentional jibe. The boom flies across and thumps the man on watch. He slumps to the deck between the cabin trunk and the portside chain plates, unconscious and bleeding furiously from a cut head.

What do you do next, Skipper? Like most of us, you would probably be scared until you had learned that basic Lifesaving First Aid is quite simple.

And that is what this chapter will show you. How simple it is: you get to work at once; no time wasted in Chinese fire drills. When you do this, order and action will supersede panic and chaos among your crew. Your injured crewman is given his best chance for quick recovery.

Any major accident anywhere, ashore or afloat, daytime or nighttime, demands attention to three basic priorities.

These are:

1. **Restore breathing.** Time is important since man suffers severe brain damage after five minutes of apnea (non-breathing).
2. **Get the victim out of further danger.**
3. **Stop serious bleeding.**

Simple, isn't it, when considered in this way? Get to your injured crewman quickly. One glance assures you he is in no further danger where he is. Do not move him. It is obvious he is bleeding; ignore that for the moment. Man can often bleed quite a while without much danger.

Note that his chest is not moving in and out; his lips, fingertips and cheeks are blue-gray. He isn't breathing.

Start mouth-to-mouth resuscitation at once (*see* Fig. 1).

1. Sweep his mouth and throat clear of blood, dentures, water, anything that obstructs the flow of air into his lungs.
2. Elevate his chin.
3. Close his nose with your thumb and forefinger.
4. Make a tight seal between his mouth and yours.
5. Take a big breath through your nose; gently blow it into his mouth and down into his lungs. His chest will rise as you do this.
6. Take your mouth away; he will exhale automatically.
7. When his lungs have pushed out all the air you blew in, give him another breath.
8. Repeat this 12 to 15 times a minute. If he is a child, put your mouth over both his mouth and nose and breathe faster (20 to 25 times a minute).
9. Do not stop until his breathing is regular. He may start suddenly, or with a series of irregular gasps. If he gasps, time your efforts between them. Let him do as much as he can, but keep assisting him until he is breathing well. How will you know? A ruddy glow will replace the blue-gray color on his lips and earlobes.

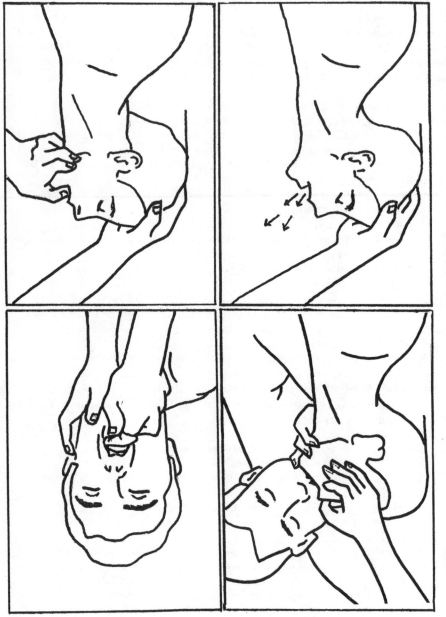

Fig. 1. **Top left:** Sweep mouth clear. **Top right:** Elevate chin. **Bottom left:** Close patient's nose, and mouth-to-mouth, blow into lungs. (**Note:** The operator's right hand should be holding the patient's nose.) **Bottom right:** Allow free expiration.

2

10. Stop then; but do not leave him unattended for the next 12 hours. Have someone stand by to assist him if he stops breathing again. This is most important if he is unconscious.

Your efforts will be more effective if you have a Resusitube and know how to use it (*see* Fig. 2). This is a plastic airway tube; one end goes in the patient's mouth and you blow on the other. There is a seal in the middle for his lips.

Your crew will be close about you and their hurt buddy and they will be greatly impressed with your prompt recognition of his non-breathing (some people think a person is dead if he is not breathing) and your skill at resuscitation. They will be standing by for your directions.

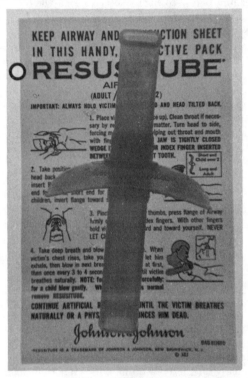

Fig. 2. Resusitube in plastic container.

Detail a sturdy fellow to stop the bleeding head. Tell him what to do between breaths as you keep up the mouth-to-mouth resuscitation.

Forget about bleeding points, pressure points and such detailed anatomy. Tell him to press down hard on whatever is bleeding. If one finger will serve—fine; if the wound is larger, he may need a whole hand. If it is bigger than that, have him stuff a gauze bandage, towel (preferably clean), or whatever is handy, into the wound and apply the pressure over this.

You will be too busy to tell him this, but you know that arterial blood pressure is rarely higher than 200 mms of Mercury; even a child can press harder than that. Direct pressure is what surgeons use in the operating room to stop bleeding.

Have him watch the blood ooze between his fingers. It slows down before it stops. Keep the pressure on ten minutes longer, then have a third crewman (who has gotten out the first-aid kit) put a tight bandage around the cut head. Chances are pretty good by this time (ten minutes after you began mouth-to-mouth and five minutes after your helper had bandaged the head) that your victim is breathing on his own.

He is "coming to"; dazed but conscious. Left unattended and apneic (not breathing) while his head was bandaged, he might never have made it. But he has, thanks to your skill and knowledge.

Now you have leisure to plan. You surely won't leave him lying there on the deck. Why not get him below to his bunk? There may be other injuries that passed unnoted in the rush to revive him. Sailors are a sturdy breed. He may insist, "I'm all right now," and try to get to his feet unaided.

Assert your authority—make him stay put. It is most embarrassing, and occurs in hospitals all the time, to overlook the injuries other than the obvious ones that attracted your attention at the time of the accident. The results of such neglect may be disastrous.

You must know how badly he is hurt. Has he hidden injury? How far away is medical help? Will you need such help, or can you handle this yourself?

We will assume he had a complete physical checkup by his physician before departure. Therefore, he has no chronic diseases that he and you do not know about.

To examine him:

1. Start at the top. He is conscious, so ask him where it hurts. His head is pretty well covered by the bandage.
2. Shine a bright flashlight into his eyes, one at a time. The pupils should be equal, and each should contract, or narrow. Unequal pupils, or one that does not contract with the light, indicates a brain concussion of a serious nature. (We will talk about head injury and the management of the unconscious patient later on.)
3. Gently move his neck, feel the entire length of his spine with your fingertips, from the base of his skull right down to, and including, his tail bone. Extreme tenderness or soreness should make you suspect a spinal injury.
4. Ask him to take a deep breath. A sharp pain in his chest may mean broken ribs. Press hard on the breastbone with your right hand and the mid-back behind with your left. This will cause pain at the site of a broken rib, just as pressure on opposite sides of a barrel springs the hoops.
5. Feel his belly gently with the flat of your hand. He may have internal injuries that won't be evident for several hours, but if his belly-wall muscles are contracted hard, and he cannot relax them when you ask him to, he probably has some such injury.
6. Finally have him move all fingers, toes, both hands, feet, ankles, wrists, arms, legs, elbows, knees, shoulders, and hips. Note if any of these hurt or are deformed or lying at an odd angle.
7. Finally you conclude:
   a. There is no serious brain damage. He is conscious, alert, knows the day

of the week, where he is, and is well oriented. His eye pupils are equal and contract alike.
b. Findings 3, 4, 5 and 6 are within normal limits.

Discussion

To the best of your knowledge he has a cut head and that is all.

While the rest of the crew are putting the injured one in his bunk, let us consider some of the commonsense and physiological reasons behind what you have done and also some other catastrophes which can switch the order of the three basic priorities. All three must be considered in any major accident but judgment is necessary to determine the order in which they are carried out.

Sometimes getting a victim away from further danger is first. If electrocution is the cause of apnea, as it may well be, do not begin mouth-to-mouth resuscitation until you get the current off, or you may join the casualty list, too.

If a severe gash cuts the brachial artery (to the arm), and a man's life is squirting away in a series of violent red gushes, the thing to do, of course, is to get a tourniquet around the arm just above the cut and twist it down until it stops the bleeding. But be sure it is spurting arterial bleeding. Look very carefully. A little blood is awesome. The usual wound will not sever a main artery; the bleeding will be a mixture of small arterial and venous bleeding, and pressure followed by bandaging will stop it.

A tourniquet too loose can make an arm or leg bleed harder. I have seen emergency patients *stop* bleeding when the tourniquet was taken off. Why?

It shut off the venous return (low pressure), but was not tight enough to close down the arterial inflow (high pressure). So if you decide on a tourniquet, twist it tight enough. Pad it well. Use a piece of line, a belt, anything sturdy enough to lay about the limb and   twist   tight. Every hour you must loosen a tourniquet long enough to make the limb below feel warm and alive again, even if the bleeding resumes while it is loosened. We will say more about the follow-up care of wounds in Chapters III and IV.

Consider a more complicated situation. You are dismasted; one of the crew is overside in a tangle of lines and stays. He is obviously in danger and must be freed up and rescued.

But is he breathing? If you spent 15 minutes or more cutting him loose and he has been apneic all that time . . . ?

If he answers your holler, you know he is conscious and breathing. But if he does not, get to him on a life line or other rig and resuscitate him while somebody else frees him up and brings him aboard.

You will both remember this with gratitude in years to come.

Many injuries produce apnea. A blow on the head, such as we have discussed, may so stun the brain that it stops driving the respiratory muscles in their proper cycles. This may be temporary; the brain may recover with a good supply of oxygen. But this is just what the non-breathing person will not get without assistance. Five minutes is the safe limit of apnea without severe brain damage or even death.

Get an extra Resusitube and keep it in your car. No ambulance ever arrives at the scene of an auto accident in time to restore a non-breathing patient; somebody else on the spot will have to do it. You? Why not? It might be someone in your own car.

Carbon monoxide exhaust from an internal combustion engine may stop the transport of oxygen from lung to brain. Hemoglobin, the red pigment in the blood cells, under normal conditions forms a loosely hung combination with oxygen in the lungs. The blood then goes to the brain or other body tissues where oxygen is easily exchanged for carbon dioxide. The body cells use the oxygen and the carbon dioxide is carried back to the lungs and exhaled. The loose combination that hemoglobin makes with oxygen in the lungs, and carbon dioxide in the tissues, makes a handy exchangeable chemical system.

Carbon monoxide from internal combustion engine fumes, on the other hand, makes a tight combination with hemoglobin that prevents oxygen pickup in the lungs and exchange for carbon dioxide in the tissues. Anoxia leads to unconsciousness; the individual may be breathing but his tissues are not getting oxygen. His location, near the fumes of an internal combustion engine with inadequate ventilation, should tell you what the trouble is. And he will be a bright *cherry red color*, formed by the combination of carbon monoxide and hemoglobin. Time is essential. He must be gotten away from the fumes by someone who can hold his breath long enough. Scuba diving gear, if nearby, can be used to rescue such a person. If he is breathing, watch him closely; if he stops, assist him. He will have an awful headache when he does come around.

This, of course, will never happen on your boat because you will always check the venting of your engine room. Even on a sailboat, this is an absolute must.

Nature is kinder to the person who bleeds than to the one in respiratory arrest or interference. Compensatory mechanisms go to work at once that can sustain life for a considerable period of time in spite of severe bleeding. Injury to body tissue—skin, muscle, bone or viscera—releases hormones into the bloodstream. These cause the blood cells and platelets to sludge (clump together), and markedly speed up clotting of the blood when it gets to the site of injury.

The blood pressure drops rapidly, too; blood loss is minimized and clots form readily under less pressure. Arteries in the extremities and outlying parts of the body constrict so that the remaining blood goes around a shorter circuit through the heart, brain, lungs and other vital organs. The heart beats faster, which helps too.

This vasoconstriction of the arteries may entirely close down a vessel in an arm or leg wound. I do not suggest that you allow nature to stop major bleeding unassisted. Do the things we have talked about earlier in this chapter, and do them promptly. But, in assessing a critical situation, remember that an injured person who is both bleeding and apneic dies of lack of oxygen rather than shortage of blood.

Emphasis is necessary because bleeding is dramatic and attracts attention, whereas apnea is rather passive.

There are other uncommon emergencies that we should mention although it is unlikely that you will encounter them.

Cardiac arrest, a sudden stopping of the heartbeat, plagues aged sailors. It is usually due to a heart attack which, in turn, is caused by a sudden lack of blood supply to the heart because of physical strain on a heart already suffering from narrowing of its own arterial blood supply by arteriosclerosis (hardening of the arteries).

1. Apnea accompanies cardiac arrest; start resuscitation by the mouth-to-mouth technique.
2. If there is no detectable pulse after you start resuscitation, give one or two sharp raps on the left mid-chest with your fist. Often this will start the heart beating.
3. When he revives control his pain (*see* Chap. IV) and insist upon absolute rest. Carry him to a bunk and make him stay there until you arrive at proper medical facilities.

Cardiac resuscitation beyond these simple measures requires sophisticated equipment, knowledge and personnel beyond the scope of this book or your experience. And even at that, ashore and with all the equipment and personnel available, the salvage rate is not great.

Penetrating chest wounds, those that make a hole through the chest wall into the pleural spaces around the lungs, are dangerous. Man's lungs hang in two vacuum sacs—the pleural cavities. He breathes by expanding his chest wall to which these sacs are attached. The pressure of the outside air forces gas down into the lungs. A hole in the chest wall destroys the vacuum (*see* Fig. 3), and though the chest wall expands, the air pressure is then equal on both the inside and outside of the lung, and the lung does not fill.

You can help this by mouth-to-mouth breathing, but you must make a much tighter seal with the victim's mouth. And you had better close the hole in the chest wall as soon as possible; put some type of dressing in or on it to seal it off. The air already in the pleural sac will be absorbed, once the hole is closed, and the lung will presently begin to work again.

At the beginning of this chapter we indicated that Lifesaving First Aid was simple enough. But now, having saved a life at some distance from medical aid, you are going to have to deal with problems that are not quite so simple.

Fortunately you will have time to consider your actions. Depending upon the availability of medical help, you are going to have to be a doctor for a varying period.

The remainder of this book is directed toward helping you decide what and how you can and cannot do until such aid is available.

A word of warning—this book will not make you a doctor; use a real doctor when one is available. Above all, do not apply what I am about to discuss with you in a foreign port where there are doctors who may not understand your language; you may think them inferior to the doctor you remember back home, but you are in their country and they must take care of you and your crew under their own laws. Doctors everywhere are striving to treat people, even strangers, to the best of their ability. You must trust them when they are available.

Treat only your own crew members and only when organized medical care is unavailable to you.

One sad example should suffice. A well-trained thoracic surgeon was on a fishing trip in a foreign port. At the end of the day's fishing, a member of another boat's crew had a cardiac arrest on the pier. This surgeon applied his skill and restored the man's heartbeat. However, the patient died a few hours later in a hospital.

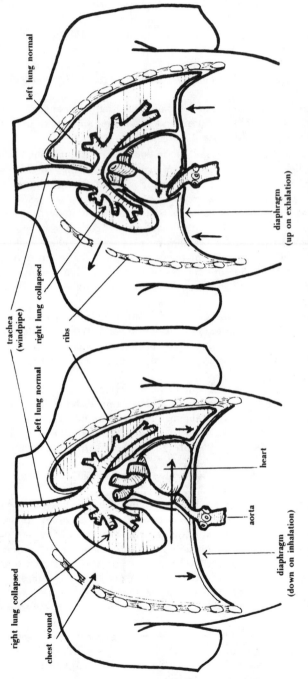

Fig. 3. Left: INHALING—Open chest wound. Note air entering chest through wound and not into right lung. Left lung normal. **Right:** EXHALING—Open chest wound. Air passes out through chest wound. Right lung has not filled with air.

left lung normal

trachea
(windpipe)

right lung collapsed

ribs

diaphragm
(up on exhalation)

left lung normal

right lung collapsed

chest wound

heart

aorta

diaphragm
(down on inhalation)

The surgeon was charged with manslaughter. He had no license to practice medicine in the particular land in which this occurred. He finally was freed, but only after a long and disagreeable experience.

I repeat—at sea, with your own crew and no help available, do all you can, as we shall try to help you do it. However, turn it over to others better qualified—even though they may not seem so to you—as soon as possible.

SUMMARY

Basic Lifesaving First Aid is easy if you know:

1. A plan prevents panic.
2. Recognize in each major catastrophe three basic priorities:
    a. Restore breathing.
    b. Get the patient out of danger.
    c. Control major bleeding.

We have discussed various situations that change the order of these priorities.

3. When the situation is under control, do a complete examination to determine the extent of the patient's injuries.
4. Physiological and other bases for the basic priorities for First Aid are discussed.
5. We have developed the concept of Second Aid, which is the care which you must exercise until such time as medical care of the proper nature is available.
6. Certain precautions in the application of advanced First Aid are discussed.

Chapter II

FRACTURES, SPRAINS AND DISLOCATIONS

You engage in a tacking duel with your nearest competitor from San Pedro Harbor Light to Point Fermin. Wind is westerly, 18 knots; you carry the 180% Genoa and make short tacks to stay out of the channel current that drives to leeward.

You come about onto the starboard tack headed out to sea; there is a yell from a winch tender. His right hand is crushed between the Genoa sheet and the Barient drum. You luff up, free his hand; he falls to the deck, pale and hurt. The right hand which he holds in his left is turning blue and swelling massively; the fourth and fifth fingers are cocked off at peculiar angles. The skin is not broken.

1. Control pain; Emperin and Codeine ½ gr. by mouth.
2. Gently straighten out the bent fingers.
3. Apply a well-padded universal arm splint with fingers in position of function (*see* Fig. 4).
4. Elevate the splinted extremity in a sling or onto the overhead of his bunk.
5. Leave fingertips exposed; loosen bandage when necessary and reapply.

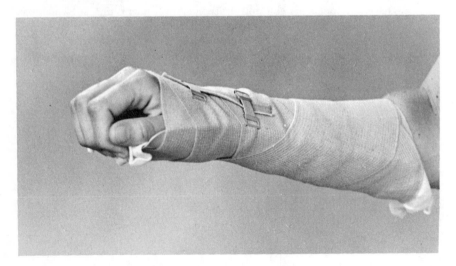

Fig. 4. Universal arm splint applied; fingers in position of function.

Crush injuries of the hand and wrist occur frequently on sailboats and damage extremely important structures.

The five steps outlined are basic treatment for all simple fractures (i.e., those that do not have an open wound extending to the broken-bone ends).

It is wise to get this patient to a hospital as soon as possible. Treatment of severe crush injuries of the hand, with or without fractures, demands sophisticated equipment and knowledge.

FOLLOW-UP CARE

If you are far out to sea and unable to get to port:

1. Continue the splint and elevation with medication.
2. Medication to control the pain.
3. After 21 days, remove the splint and gently move the uninjured fingers. This will reduce the swelling somewhat in the rest of the hand.
4. Replace the splint but leave uninjured fingers unbound so they may move.
5. Over the course of the next two weeks, gradually increase the motion of the hand and fingers.
6. When movement no longer hurts, remove the cast.

Do not worry about whether there is a fracture. This treatment described is equally effective for crush injury without broken bones.

SPLINTS

Simple fractures are treated by immobilization in a splint until the broken-bone ends heal together. A splint is a simple machine long enough and strong enough to immobilize the broken bone, one joint above and one joint below the fracture. It must be well padded to protect the skin and bony parts from pressure sores. Splint-padding material or liner is not expensive and does not require much storage space (*see* Fig. 5). If you lack a supply of cast liner, material such as strips of cloth, towels, etc., furnish a good substitute.

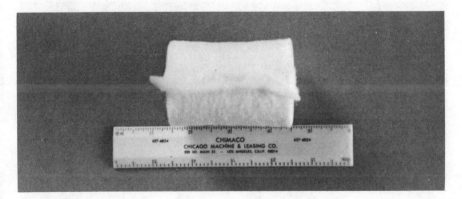

Fig. 5. Cast liner.

The best splints for use on shipboard are the cardboard type which stow flat and are folded up for use. Two or three of these lengths suitable for the arms and legs of your crew members, plus the universal hand splint, will care for your needs for a cruise of any length.

Pneumatic splints also stow flat, and after being applied to the fractured extremity, are inflated. It is important to do this only with mouth pressure, otherwise it may stop circulation.

Traction splints are also available and popular with ambulance services but these require more stowage space and are difficult to apply correctly. The traction is an advantage but the hazards on shipboard outweigh the advantages, in my opinion.

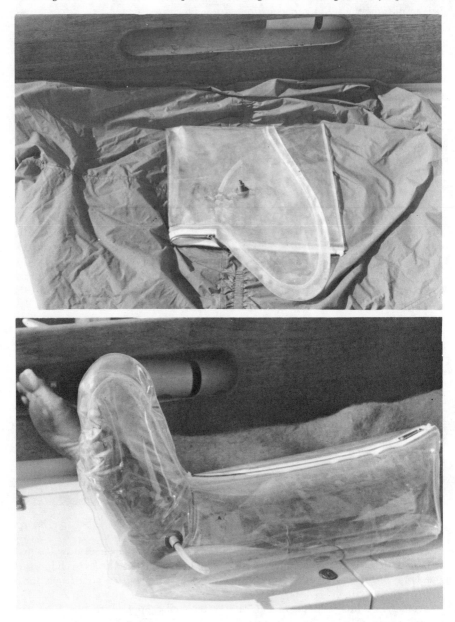

Fig. 6. Top: Pneumatic leg splint folded for storage. **Bottom:** Pneumatic leg splint applied.

If you lack prefabricated splints, many materials aboard may be employed. Use your imagination: Swab handles, winch handles, heavy pillows, sail battens, or navigational charts folded to the requisite stiffness can be used satisfactorily.

I recently saw an excellent splint fashioned from four segments of a broom handle that enabled a camper to bring his wife comfortably 400 miles out of the desert to the hospital. He was a certified public accountant by trade but proudly designed and created this splint for his wife's broken knee.

SIMPLE FRACTURES

A member of your crew steps into an open hatch, falls forward and catches his left mid-leg on the hatch combing. There is a loud crack; he lands on the deck with his leg angled awkwardly and exquisitely painful. He cannot stand on it; the effort is agonizing. The skin is unbroken.

1. Examine the leg gently; cut away his trousers to get a good look at it.
2. Feel his shin. You will probably find the edges of the broken bone.
3. Let him lie unless he has fallen into an inaccessible position. If he has, wrap the broken leg firmly to the uninjured one with an Ace bandage before you move him to a convenient spot to work on him.
4. Give him Demerol; 100 mgms (2 cc) by injection (*see* Fig. 7).
5. Wipe first with antiseptic. Inject 20 cc 1% Xylocaine into fracture site.
6. Straighten out the right, unbroken leg with the ankle held to a right angle.
7. Sight through the right great toe to the center of the right kneecap. This is the normal weight-bearing line.
8. Brace yourself; take a firm grip fore and aft on the left ankle.
9. Have assistant hold the injured man under the armpits.
10. Pull the broken leg slowly out straight; this is traction. Be steady; watch the broken part. Do not force the bone ends to poke out through the skin—this would compound the fracture.
11. Slowly bring the broken leg into the proper weight-bearing line.
12. Traction should make the injured leg feel better.
13. Your assistant pulls from above; this makes countertraction.
14. You feel the bones move into an end-on-end position. Keep the traction on and slowly lift the leg. Let a third helper slide a folded-up and padded cardboard splint into place. This must be long enough to go from toes to well above the knee and fit snugly.
15. Wrap the leg and splint firmly together with an Ace bandage. Leave toes exposed.
16. Now very slowly let off the traction (your pull) and countertraction (the helper's pull under the armpits).
17. Two of you carry him to his bunk. Detail another man to manage the splinted leg. Coordinate your movements.
18. Elevate the splinted leg.
19. Continue pain control with Demerol, as needed. If you use Demerol or codeine for a few days, you will have to give a laxative because these drugs are constipating.
20. Watch his toes. If they become very swollen, blue, numb, and at the same time, painful, the cast is too tight.

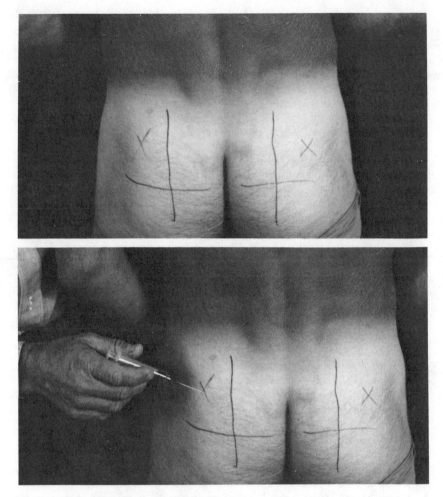

Fig. 7. Top: Area for intramuscular injection—upper outer quadrant of either buttock.
Bottom: Angle of needle insertion. **(Continued on next page.)**

21. Reapply the traction and countertraction.
22. Unwrap the bandage around the splint, including the final turn. Hold traction; wait for toes to "come alive" and feel warm.
23. Rewrap the splint, then let off the traction.
24. Do this as often as necessary; the broken leg will hurt at the site of the fracture. This is different from the pain of a splint that is too tight.
25. You will want to get outside help; this fracture requires a minimum of three months to heal. Meanwhile, maintain splint, control pain and watch the circulation in the toes.

Handle fractures of the elbow and shoulder differently. The location of important nerves and blood vessels close to these bones makes it imperative that

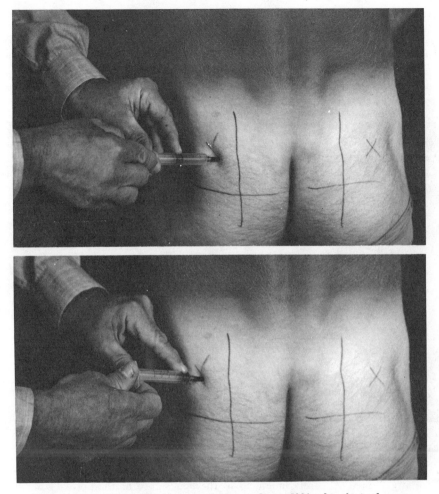

Fig. 7 (continued). Top: Needle inserted; plunger drawn. If blood is obtained, move needle—it is in a vein. **Bottom:** Injection completed.

minimum efforts be undertaken to line up or reduce the fracture. Such injuries should be gently straightened out so you will not drive a broken bone end through an artery or nerve.

Fractures of the forearm (between the elbow and wrist) often produce a striking deformity. It is safe to straighten these enough to apply a splint handily, but watch the bone ends; never compound a fracture by pushing the ends through the skin. Be gentle; apply steady non-jerking traction.

The hand splint is useful for forearm fractures. After the splint is applied, the limb can be brought to a right angle at the elbow and held in a sling around the neck. Then, additional support can be offered from elbow to upper arm.

Fractures of the arm (shoulder to elbow) are usually not remarkably deformed.

They present a problem for splinting because it is difficult to immobilize the joint above (i.e., the shoulder).

It is best to splint an arm fracture with the elbow at a right angle and a cardboard splint applied. This extends from the wrist, around the elbow and as high as possible on the arm. A sling will help and if immobilization is still inadequate as noted by severe, increasing pain at the fracture site, the arm and forearm may be bound to the chest wall. Usually, this is not necessary.

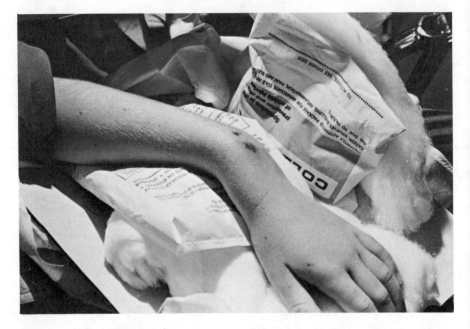

Fig. 8. Simple fracture, both bones of forearm—angulation at mid third.

Fractures of the wrist and ankle are splinted without traction. If severe deformity is present, gentle moulding to the appearance of the normal side will help.

As in all fractures, rough, irregular movements are forbidden. If there is a question in your mind, it is better to splint the broken bone in the position in which you find it. You will thus do no further harm. This is a prime principle of all medical practice.

SPINAL FRACTURES

Dr. Arthur Davis, a fine orthopedic surgeon and racing sailor, devised the modern method of reducing broken backs.

He cut a ring life preserver in half and fastened the two halves together to make a rounded splint over which he stretched the patient's broken back. This extension brought the cracked vertebrae back into line and a cast was then applied.

This principle is still used, although the equipment has been changed.

The danger from spinal fractures is injury to the spinal cord, resulting in paralysis.

Such damage may occur at the time of accident. In this case, not much can be done about it. It may occur following improper handling after the spine is broken. This is a preventable tragedy.

Acute forward bending (flexion) causes most spinal fractures. Cervical spine fractures commonly occur as a result of diving into shallow water; the head strikes the bottom and the full weight of the body bends it forward.

This type of injury and extreme tenderness over the neck bones on the gentlest feeling (under no circumstances allow the patient's head to bend forward when you examine him) would cause you to suspect a neck (cervical) fracture.

There is rarely any apparent angulation of a broken neck. Minimal movement laterally will cause pain at the site of the broken vertebra.

If the patient is paralyzed (cannot move his feet or hands), the spinal cord is damaged. Care for him as described in the section about the Unconscious Patient (*see* Chap. VIII).

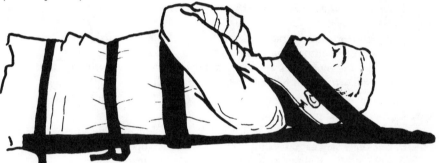

Fig. 9. Suitable splint for fractured spine.

If you suspect a cervical fracture and there is no paralysis:

1. Do not move the patient.
2. Sit above him, with his head between your legs.
3. Put one hand on either side of his jaw; pull gently but firmly up without bending his head forward.
4. Now have someone else give him an injection of Demerol (75-100 mgms or 1½ cc) if he is in pain.
5. Hold traction and have your assistant slide a board under his neck and upper back. A crib board is good for this purpose. A hatch cover may be used; any rigid structure that extends from the back of his head to his mid-back behind.
6. If the board is narrow, wrap a bandage about his head to hold his neck firmly in place (*see* Fig. 9). If the board is wider, pad either side of his head out to the bandage.
7. Slowly release traction.
8. Have two or three persons lift him so his trunk and the splint remain level.
9. Carry him level to his bunk and put him there, board and all.
10. Keep him flat and splintered until you get to help. He can stay that way as long as necessary.
11. Control pain with continuing medication.

Should a diving accident occur and the patient still be in the water, it would not be possible to exert traction on his neck. Swim alongside him and bend his head backward, gently (extension). Then float a board under his neck and back and fasten him to it firmly before you bring him out of the water.

But wait a minute! Did you check his breathing? Did he need to be resuscitated? Remember, this comes first.

Fractures of the lower (thoracic and lumbar) spine are rare injuries on shipboard. These are also caused by forceful flexion. Management is similar—rigid splinting before movement and control of pain. Traction for these injuries is rarely possible on shipboard.

BROKEN NOSES

Broken noses are not serious unless they bleed too much, too long. All broken noses bleed, but most of them stop within an hour or so.

1. Apply pressure. Pinch the nostrils together with a hot (*not cold*) rag, or just your fingers.
2. If this does not work, take the forceps from the First-Aid Kit and pack some cotton into the bleeding nostril.
3. If bleeding continues and the patient is alarmed, Emperin and Codeine, ½ gr., will often quiet him and aid to stop bleeding.

If all these measures fail and bleeding is continuing at a profuse rate, you will have to make a nasal pack:

4. If you have not given an analgesic (Demerol 75 mgms), do so now.
5. Get the Foley catheter in its prepackaged envelope.
6. Fill the little balloon with 4 cc of air to test it; then deflate it.
7. Decide which nostril is bleeding.
8. Sit your patient up with firm support behind his head.
9. Lubricate the Foley catheter with Vaseline, salad oil, or 3-in-One, etc.
10. Pass the catheter into the bleeding nostril; it will encounter resistance, but press firmly and gently on.
11. Sudden end to the resistance tells you the tip of the catheter has passed into the nasopharynx (chamber behind the nose).
12. Inflate the balloon in the Foley catheter with 4 cc of air (or 30 cc, depending upon which size of catheter you have—it is plainly marked).
13. Pull catheter forward firmly; the balloon will close off the backside of the nasal chamber. All of the bleeding should be coming out of the front of the nose. If there is any blood running down behind (ask the patient), pull the catheter forward more vigorously.
14. Anchor catheter firmly to the forehead with several strips of adhesive. The pressure will be uncomfortable; if it is not, you do not have it tight enough.
15. Pack nostril in front of catheter balloon with cotton.

You now have the nasal chamber packed fore and aft and bleeding will be limited to that small space.

You will need to give Demerol freely (100 mgms or 1½ cc every three hours) because this pack is misery. Add Valium 5 mgms (a tranquilizer) by injection every 4-6 hours if your broken-beaked crewman cannot tolerate the pack with Demerol alone.

16. In 12 hours, remove the cotton from the nostril; if blood flows, repack the nostril and do not disturb the catheter. (But, if blood is running down the throat behind, trim it a bit tighter to the forehead.)
17. Check every 12 hours. If there is no bleeding when cotton is removed from the nostril, wait four hours.
18. When you are sure bleeding has stopped, deflate the balloon of the catheter and *very slowly and gently draw it out.*

Final word of warning: Do not be in any hurry to remove the catheter. It is difficult to replace.

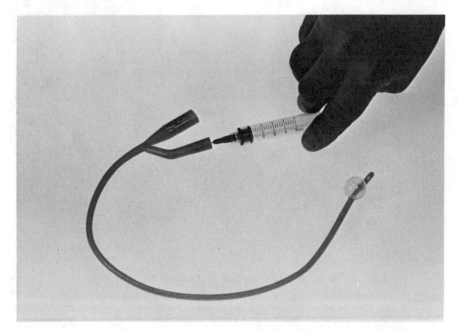

Fig. 10. Foley (inlying) catheter: method of testing balloon before insertion. Air injection.

OTHER COMMON FRACTURES

Fractures of the collarbone are caused by a sidewise fall onto the shoulder. They cause immediate local pain and tenderness. The injured individual cannot raise his arm beyond 90° from his side without severe pain.

Feel the uninjured clavicle and then the suspected one. Run your fingers along from breastbone to shoulder. Seek irregularity, swelling, tenderness, or even jagged bone ends beneath the skin (*see* Fig. 11).

Reduce a fractured clavicle in the following manner:

1. Give Demerol 75-100 mgms by injection.
2. Seat the patient on a stool and stand directly behind him.
3. Inject local anesthesia (10 cc of 1% Xylocaine) into the fracture site.
4. Have one assistant on each side raise each arm as high and as far backward as possible.

5. The operator grasps the top of each shoulder from the back to front; put your right knee between the patient's shoulder blades. Pull hard.

6. When reduction is accomplished as determined by the movements of the bones and a snap, fashion a heavy figure-of-eight bandage running under both armpits across the back of the neck (*see* Fig. 12). In front, pass them over the bony prominences of the shoulder, not under the armpit.

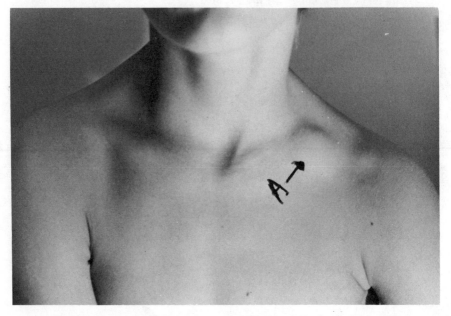

Fig. 11. Fracture mid third left clavicle (collarbone). Tender swelling at A.

7. When the reduction and splinting are accomplished, if an arm becomes numb or begins to swell a great deal, release the bandage; it is cutting off the axillary artery to the arm. A fractured clavicle, even if unreduced, will heal. Do not risk loss of blood flow to the arm.

If the reduction is unsuccessful or if the patient cannot tolerate the figure-of-eight bandage as described, put the arm in a sling.

Pelvic fractures are caused by severe crush injuries. A sailor caught between dock and boat or having heavy gear fall across the pelvis can suffer such an injury.

Pressure on the lateral sides of the pelvis over the two iliac crests, pressure from front to back from the pubic region to the lower lumbar region, which causes sharp pain in a localized area, suggests a pelvic fracture.

The treatment for such fractures is rest in bed and Demerol or Emperin and Codeine.

One complication which may occur in a severe pelvic fracture that can be helped on shipboard is interference with urination. Swelling around a broken pelvic bone near the bladder may obstruct urine flow.

If the patient with suspected pelvic fracture is unable to void for a period of eight to ten hours, it will be necessary to pass a catheter (*see* Chap. VI for technique). Leave it inlying and start Azo-Gantrisin 0.5 gm four times a day, with a glass of water at each dose, as long as the catheter is in place.

The Colles fracture (named after the 17th century Dublin surgeon) occurs at the wrist. It is caused by a fall on the outstretched hand.

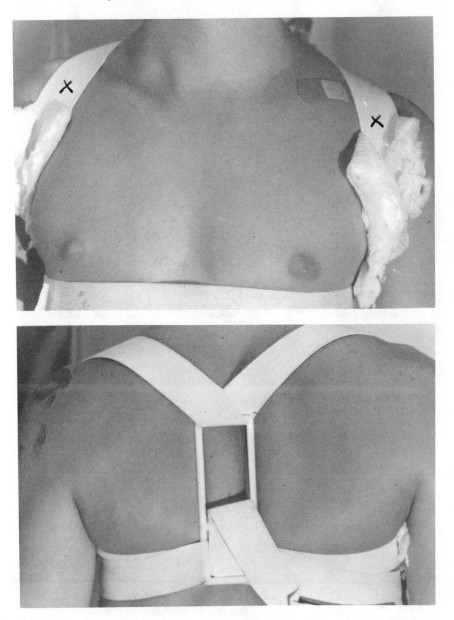

Fig. 12. Top: Front view clavicular splint. Note pressure is on bony points of shoulder, X and X. Band-Aid covers site of local anesthesia injection. Bottom: Rear view clavicular splint. Same pressure can be held with heavy figure-of-eight bandage.

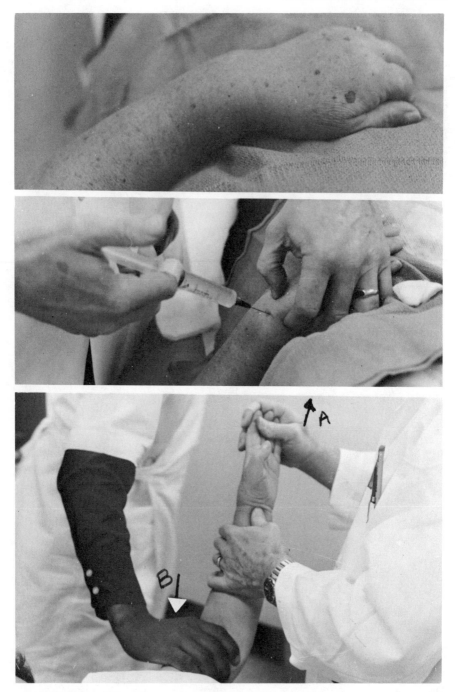

Fig. 13. Top: Broken wrist; Colles fracture. **Center:** Injection of local anesthesia into fracture site of broken wrist. **Bottom:** traction (A), countertraction (B); reduction of broken wrist.

There is the so-called "Silver Fork" deformity (*see* Fig. 13). Pain and inability to move the wrist accompany it.

Though it is difficult to maintain this fracture after reduction, it will do little harm to attempt the following:

1. Demerol 75-100 mgms (1½ cc) by injection.
2. After antiseptic wipe, inject 10 cc 1% Xylocaine into fracture site.
3. Assistant applies countertraction to arm just above the elbow (*see* Fig. 13).
4. Operator holds patient's hand in his opposite hand (patient's left to operator's right, or vice versa).
5. Operator exerts steady, firm, straight traction while assistant maintains steady countertraction. Do not jerk but do not be afraid to pull.
6. When bones move at fracture site, cock the hand up sharply, put thumbs (operator's) across lower ends of broken bones and slide them down into place. Straighten out wrist.
7. Reduction will be accompanied by movement of bones at the fracture site and often a grating sound or click.
8. Hold wrist until universal arm splint is strapped firmly to wrist and hand.
9. Follow-up care as for other fractures.

Fractured toes usually occur with a stubbed toe—a barefoot sailor, a deck cleat, a dark night. They are not fatal but may be very painful.

Splint by taping them firmly to adjoining toes. Wear a shoe until barefoot walking is painless.

SPRAINS

Thumbs, fingers and ankles are frequently sprained; wrists and necks less often at sea. A thumb bent too far backward stretches or tears the ligaments that support the joint. Often a small fracture accompanies it.

If such injury to the thumb or finger is accompanied by great pain and huge swelling that is aggravated by any attempt to move the part, treat it as a fracture. Give medication for pain (Demerol or Emperin and Codeine) and apply the universal arm or other splint (with the fingers in the position of function).

Follow-up care keeps the splint in place, loosening it when necessary, for a minimum of three weeks.

It is safe enough to remove the splint for a trial of motion after three weeks. If this is successful, it suggests a mild sprain and may safely be removed. If pain persists, then the splint must be reapplied.

A sprained ankle without accompanying fracture need not put its owner out of action. You can find out in this way:

1. Seat the injured with calf of leg resting on support, injured foot and ankle sticking beyond.
2. Shave ankle and leg to mid-calf.
3. Paint the foot, ankle and leg to the mid-calf with compound tincture of benzoin.
4. Run a light sheet around the great toe. Have patient hold both ends and maintain the ankle at a 90° angle.
5. Cut a strip of 1-inch adhesive tape long enough to reach from six inches above the ankle inside the leg, under the foot and up to the same level on the outside of the leg. This is a stirrup.

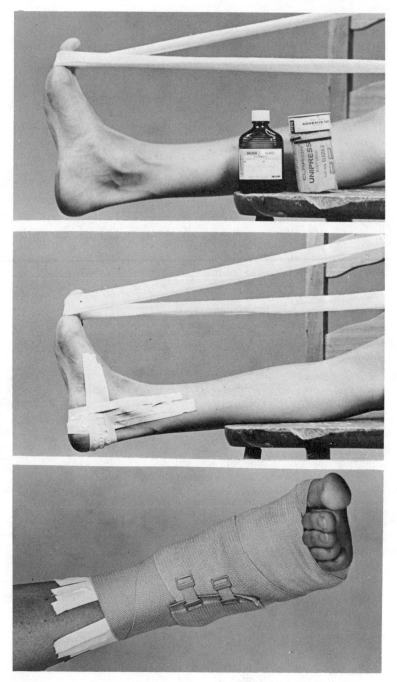

Fig. 14. Top: Position and supplies for ankle strapping—therapeutic test for possible fracture. **Center:** Alternate anchors and stirrups. **Bottom:** Completed bandage; ready for test of weight bearing.

6. Mould stirrup smoothly down the inside of the ankle (after the benzoin is dry and sticky). Run it smoothly under the foot to the outside of the leg; pull up and stick it down.
7. Cut another strip of 1-inch tape long enough to reach from the base of the great toe, around the ankle horizontally and to the base of the fifth toe. This is an anchor.
8. Alternate anchors and stirrups until the ankle is covered.
9. When weave is finished, wrap an Ace bandage over the tape firmly.
10. The smoother the tape, the more comfortable the bandage.
11. Now have the patient stand up on his good foot and put weight gradually on the taped ankle.
12. If he can begin to walk about with slight discomfort, he has a mild sprain. Take him off the sick list but send him to light duty. If weight-bearing hurts a lot, he has a bad sprain with torn ligaments and/or a fracture. Put a cardboard ankle splint over the adhesive strapping and consign him to his bunk for three weeks or the end of the cruise, whichever comes first.
13. If he can walk at first, but over the course of 12 hours the pain becomes more severe do the same as step No. 12.

You have just completed a therapeutic test. You lose no time because the boot will help the splint to hold the ankle if he cannot walk.

This dressing was devised by a British Army surgeon to keep soldiers with sprained ankles active. It will do this for sailors, too. Note that no tape passes around the ankle. If it swells, loosen the overlying Ace bandage and reapply it.

More words about sprained ankles. In a severe emergency (not to win a sailboat race) when every crew member may be needed or each may need to be as agile as possible for his own rescue, you may, if possible under these conditions, render the ankle usable by controlling the pain.

Draw 5-10 cc of 1% Xylocaine into a sterile syringe. Wipe the ankle with antiseptic; find the tenderest spot and inject it. Move the needle about the ankle joint until all painful areas are injected.

This should be reserved for an extreme situation since it will allow the individual to use and further damage a sprained ankle.

DISLOCATIONS

Finger dislocations are the most common jumped-out joints you will see. The diagnosis is obvious to anyone. What you cannot tell is whether there is a fracture as well.

Get to a finger dislocation within a few moments. It will be numb for a bit. A straight pull pops it back painlessly. (Remove all finger rings at once; cut if necessary). After you relocate a dislocated finger, apply a splint in the position of function (for one finger). Leave it on for 14 days at least to allow the strained joint ligaments to heal.

Another common dislocation is the shoulder. After a twisting force, you will note:

1. An immobilized, painful arm held tightly to the side of the chest.
2. Severe pain throughout the whole shoulder area.

3. A depression over the shoulder joint as compared to the normal one on the other side.

You may safely reduce this as follows:

1. Give Demerol 100 mgms (2 cc) by injection.
2. Allow 40 minutes for the patient to relax, reclining on a bunk in any comfortable position.
3. Turn him onto his belly. Place the good arm under his forehead and let the dislocated shoulder hang out over the edge of the bunk.
4. Apply traction steadily on the arm down towards the deck.
5. Increase pull gradually. If you aggravate the pain, the muscles will tighten down and defeat your attempted reduction.
6. Be in no hurry. If you get tired of pulling, have the victim hold 5-10 pounds in his hand (a bucket of water, etc.).
7. It will reduce "all at once" usually with an audible snap.
8. The relief from pain will be great.
9. Apply a sling and bandage the arm to the side of his chest with elbow at a right angle.
10. Keep him splinted thus for three weeks. Then gradually begin motion.
11. Have him bend forward with injured shoulder and arm falling free, and swing hand in everwidening circles. Start gradually and extend this as fast as possible daily until full range of shoulder motion returns (circumduction exercises).

SUMMARY

Basic treatment of all simple fractures (those without a wound in continuity with broken bone ends) is:

1. Control pain.
2. Apply padded splint.
3. Bandage with moderate pressure.
4. Elevate the splinted extremity.
5. Watch splinted extremity for impaired circulation.

The above is good treatment for crush wounds of the extremities without an open wound, as well.

Types of splints are discussed.

Details of management of a broken leg are presented.

Fractures that can be reduced with reasonable safety if gently done are:

1. Leg.
2. Forearm.
3. Arm.

Fractures that generally should be splinted as they lie are:

1. Elbow.
2. Shoulder.

Spinal fractures are discussed.

Nasal fractures with severe bleeding to control are discussed.

Other common fractures are discussed.

Treatment of common sprains (thumb, fingers, ankle) is detailed.

Dislocations of fingers and shoulder are detailed.

Discussion of fracture healing is at the end of Chapter III.

Chapter III

COMPOUND FRACTURES, WOUNDS AND AMPUTATIONS

COMPOUND FRACTURES

A sudden squall hits the *Sea Witch* at 0400 hours on a Monday halfway between Tarawa and Penryhn in the Gilbert Islands. Before you douse the mizzen staysail, it pulls a pad eye from the deck. The deck watch ducks and throws up a hand. It takes the full force of the flying block.

The sailor falls to the deck aft the cockpit, his left hand torn and bleeding. Bone ends poke through the skin. He sits up, inspects his ruined hand, unbelieving.

1. Wrap the hand firmly in a suitable splint (cardboard or other) on the spot (*see* Fig. 4).
2. Assist him to his bunk.
3. Give him 100 mgms of Demerol by injection.
4. Prepare the following:
   Three quarts of water boiled 20 minutes, cooled with cover on; Phisohex; elastic bandages; gauze squares.
5. Scrub your hands five minutes at galley sink with Phisohex and fresh water. Rinse with part of the sterile water.
6. Remove the splint you applied in step No. 1 then press gauze squares firmly over wound with left hand (*see* (Fig. 15).
7. Scrub the skin around the wound with Phisohex and sterile water. Hold gauze in right hand. Have assistant pour sterile water onto gauze and wound as needed.
8. Shave the area around the wound.
9. Now remove the gauze in left hand from the wound. Throw it away. Inject Xylocaine 1% into wound surfaces.
10. Take fresh gauze and more Phisohex. Scrub inside the wound, including broken bone ends, thoroughly. Get it clean; remove chips of loose bone and dirt. Leave bone fragments that are attached.
11. Rinse three times with sterile water.
12. Press fresh dry gauze onto wound until bleeding from the washup stops (4-10 minutes).
13. Observe the patient's right uninjured hand; mould the broken bones of the left hand into a similar configuration. Injection of Xylocaine 1% (15-20 cc) into the wound edges and about the broken bones will make this less painful.
14. Squeeze a generous dollop of Bacitracin or Neosporin ointment into the wound.
15. Place sterile gauze over the whole wound.
16. Apply an Ace or other bandage firmly over the gauze.
17. Apply a universal hand splint with the fingers in the position of function (*see* Fig. 4) and secure it with a second firm bandage.
18. Elevate the splinted arm above the patient's head.
19. Give ampicillin 500 mgms by mouth.

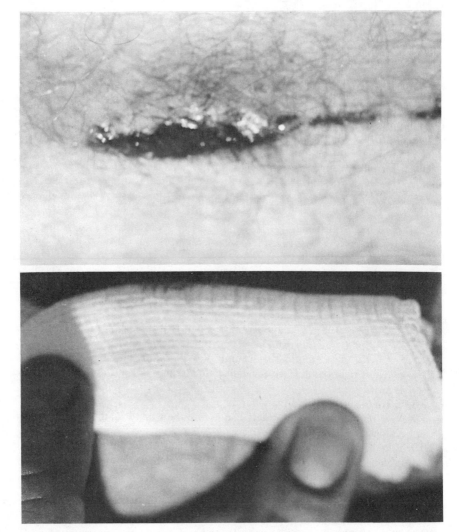

Fig. 15. Top: Deep leg wound. Bottom: Wound packed with sterile gauze—leg around
wound scrubbed and shaved. (Continued on next page.)

This completes the primary definitive treatment of a compound fracture, i.e., a
fracture with an open wound in continuity with the broken bone ends. This case
involves the wrist but the treatment applies to any compound fracture. Should a leg
be involved, after the washup and dressing are applied and before you splint the
extremity, it will be advisable to reduce the broken-bone ends to an end-on-end
position by traction and countertraction. See description for simple fractures in
Chapter II.

Follow-up care of the compound fracture:

1. Maintain the splinted position.
2. Control pain with injections of Demerol 75-100 mgms (1½-2 cc) every four
   hours as necessary.

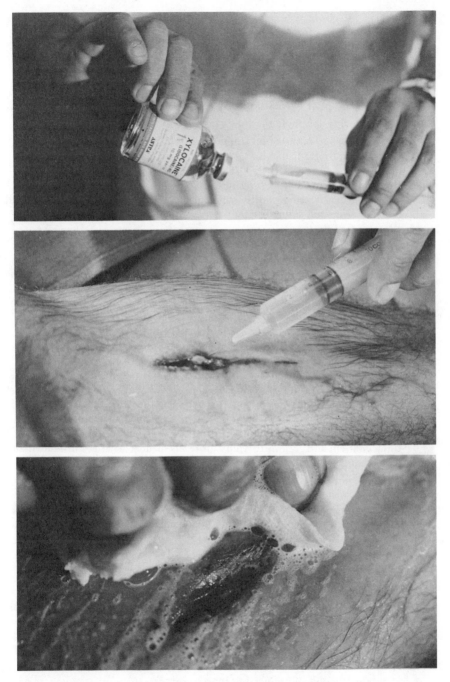

Fig. 15 (continued). Top: Drawing local anesthesia from multiple-dose vial. Wipe rubber stopper with antiseptic before puncture. **Center:** Injection of local anesthesia to numb wound. **Bottom:** Scrub-out of wound. May now be closed or packed open.

3. Prevent infection with ampicillin (or other antibiotic) by mouth 250 mgms every four hours for ten days.
4. Change the wound dressing as often as necessary, i.e., when soaked with blood and serum; preferably before it begins to smell. This interval may be hours, days, or (in cool climates) several days.
5. Observe fingertips every four hours for coldness and numbness; loosen bandages if splint becomes too tight. Remember to loosen both bandages.

To change dressing, assemble the following:
1. Sterile water; 20-minute boil and cool with lid on.
2. Give Demerol 100 mgms by injection if patient has had none for past two hours.
3. Remove and discard dirty dressings.
4. Wash skin and wound gently with Phisohex and sterile water. Remove all crusted serum and exudate.
5. Rinse wound gently.
6. Cover with Bacitracin or Neosporin ointment.
7. Apply clean gauze and a bandage over the wound.
8. It is better to wrap wound bandage outside the one holding the splint to the part. Then you may expose the wound without loosening the splint. This maintains reduction.
9. You have to care for the patient, too. A broken leg ties him to his bunk for the rest of the cruise. He may hobble painfully to the head with help but a bottle and pail are simpler. A bedpan is a handy item. You may lug one thousands of miles and never use it but if you have space, take one along.
10. Codeine and Demerol are constipating drugs. Give a good laxative such as Milk of Magnesia if your patient goes a day or two without a bowel movement or he may develop a fecal impaction which he cannot pass. It will have to be removed by hand.
11. Narcotic drugs plus inactivity and pain may make urination difficult. Force fluids and encourage him to void before his bladder becomes distended and too uncomfortable.

Often a man will be able to void if he can touch the deck with just one foot.

If he becomes distended (12-18 hours), you may have to catheterize him (*see* Chap. VI). Do not be in any hurry. He will void spontaneously before he ruptures his bladder, although the agony of waiting may be more than you and he can bear.

Discussion of Fractures

Basic treatment for all fractures is:
1. Immediate reduction of the part to normal alignment. If the patient is in an inaccessible spot, bind the broken limb firmly to the sound one, then move him to a better location.
2. Splint the broken bone ends plus one joint above and one joint below, when anatomically possible.
3. Maintain immobilization until healing is complete.
4. If fracture is compound, splint in deformed position first, cleanse wound to prevent bone infection, then remove the first splint. Reduce the fracture and reapply the splint. Leave the skin wound open.

It has been known for centuries that immediately following a fracture the tissues are in a state of local "shock." Pain is nil. This period lasts a few minutes. Shortly pain begins and nearby muscles set into spasm which locks the broken bone ends wherever they lie.

There is considerable bleeding, too, at the fracture site from the marrow cavities of the broken bones and from injury to the surrounding soft parts. A hematoma (blood clot) develops. Swelling and further stiffening and immobilization of the tissue follow.

Reduction will be more likely to succeed if it is done while the part is numb and before spasm and swelling develop. After reduction spasm helps to hold the reduction. Paul Colona, a well-known orthopedic surgeon, has said:

> "The use of immediate emergency traction for simple, i.e., non compound, fractures
> if universally adapted would constitute the biggest single advance in the treatment of
> fractures in the present generation."

He refers to lay persons' efforts at the site of an accident.

Firm, steady pull on any fractured extremity that draws it into a normal position like the opposite uninjured limb will never do harm.

Make an exception for compound fracture. If reduced before washup, the bone ends carry dirt into the wound.

Be swift with a compound fracture. You may finish the washup before the numb period ends. If not you can surely wash up and splint in an hour; the swelling usually does not appear for two hours or sometimes longer.

Local anesthesia, 1% Xylocaine (30-40 cc) injected into the fracture site under aseptic precautions, will relieve pain and help in the washup and reduction.

It is a working rule among surgeons that there is no timetable for healing of fractures. This is determined by X-ray examination at regular intervals. So, lacking X-rays, you will maintain the splint on a major bone fracture until help arrives. A broken leg, for example, requires from three to five months or even longer to heal.

Fractures heal by spanning the gap between broken bone ends with an interlacing network of fine fibrils derived from the local hematoma. Delicate cells (fibroblasts) creep out along this network to form soft scar tissue. A second type of cells (osteoblasts) deposit calcium that hardens the scar into callus. It is this solid callus which welds the bone ends firmly together. The whole process takes several weeks or months.

Such tissue growth is easily interrupted by movement of bone ends that tear the latticework of fibrils much as a spider's web is torn by movement of anchoring bushes.

Infection at the fracture site replaces the tissue growth with a different type of activity; one aimed to destroy the invading bacteria. All healing stops until the infection is destroyed and eliminated with the formation of pus.

Strict immobilization and absence of infection promote prompt healing of any fracture. If, on the other hand, the healing process is delayed by undue mobility or infection, subsequent repair becomes prolonged and difficult. Bone grafts and other surgical operations are often needed.

If you can prevent infection and maintain immobilization of a fracture on shipboard, you will save your shipmate a good deal of suffering and disability when the doctors take over.

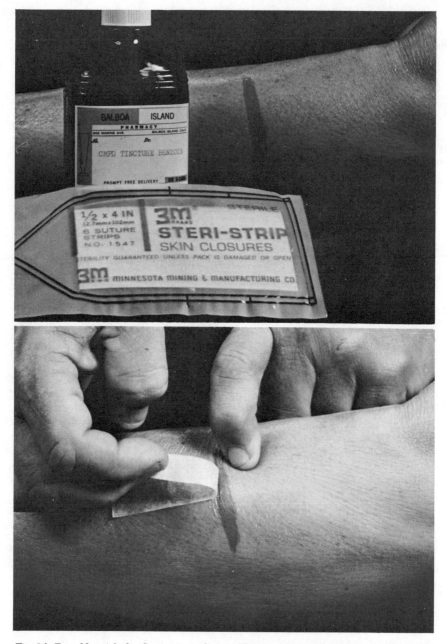

Fig. 16. Top: Materials for Steri-strip technique. **Bottom:** Steri-strip technique. **(Continued on next page.)**

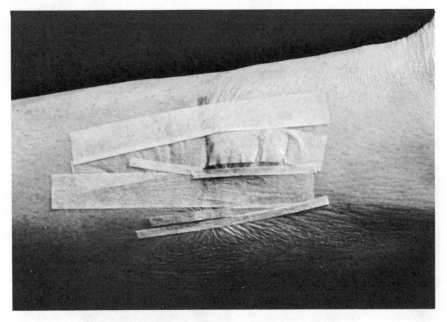

Fig. 16 (continued). Completed Steri-strip closure.

WOUNDS

Wounds, like Shakespeare's "Cleopatra," are of infinite variety. Size, location, cause and hazard to life and limb may vary. A knife cut on the finger is a wound; so is a leg ripped off by a shark's teeth. The latter at first glance seems more serious but sailors have survived shark bite while other sailors have died from apparently simple lacerations.

The basic treatment of wounds is:

1. Stop major bleeding.
2. Wash up the wound.
3. Close the skin only. Make no attempt to close tendons, nerves or other deep-lying structures.
4. Bandage.
5. Change bandage as necessary.
6. Remove sutures when wound is healed.
7. If infection develops, remove all skin closure (Steri-strips or sutures). Spread the wound widely.
8. Apply moist warm compresses to infected wound.
9. Give systemic antibiotics when indicated.

To close a wound with Steri-strips:

1. After washup (as for compound fractures) and control of bleeding, dry wound edges thoroughly.
2. Paint both edges of wound with compound tincture of benzoin.

3. When dry, stick a Steri-strip firmly to one skin margin. Pull the wound together and stick strip to opposite skin edge (*see* Fig. 16).
4. Repeat until wound is well covered with Steri-strips.
5. You may substitute adhesive tape butterflies, store-bought or homemade.
6. Bandage firmly over Steri-strips.

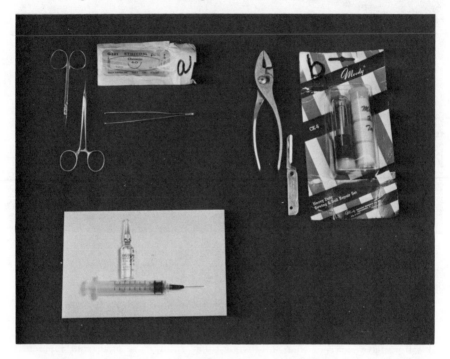

Fig. 17. A) Surgical sewing kit. B) Available substitutes. No substitutes for syringe and local anesthesia.

To suture (sew up) a wound, assemble:

1. Prepackaged silk or nylon, 2-0 or 3-0 sutures, swedged onto curved cutting needles.
2. Needle holder—sterile, prepackaged.
3. Scissors.
4. Toothed tissue forceps.
5. Sterile, prepackaged 4" x 4" gauze squares.
6. 10 cc hypodermic syringe and No. 21 or No. 22 needle, sterile, prepackaged.
7. Xylocaine 1% ampules (5 cc) or multiple-dose vial of 50 ml.

This is ideal. If your First-Aid Kit is incomplete, substitute:

1. Sail or other sewing kit for swedged-on sutures.
2. Pliers for needle holder.
3. Razor blade or knife for scissors to cut sutures (thread).
4. Clean cloths, 4" x 4" for sterile gauze squares.

5. There is no satisfactory substitute for hypodermic needles or Xylocaine (*see* Fig. 17).
6. If you are unable to inject local anesthesia, sew without it. Emperin + Codeine ½ gr. by mouth, plus other handy internally ingested analgesics, will make the process bearable for the victim.

All unsterile (i.e., not prepackaged) instruments and supplies can be sterilized by boiling for 20 minutes in a covered pan.

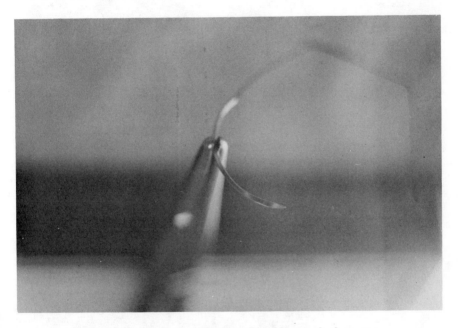

Fig. 18A. Placement of needle in needle holder—swedged-on suture.

To sterilize previously opened prepackaged plastic syringes or instruments, do not heat. Soak in alcohol for one hour; heat melts the plastic.

Details of wound suture:

1. Wash up as described for compound fracture.
2. Inject wound edges with local anesthesia as shown.
3. Do not inject more than 50 cc (ml) of 1% Xylocaine.
4. Apply constant pressure over gauze to stop bleeding caused by the washup and injection of local anesthetic (four to ten minutes).
5. Check anesthesia; touch sensation remains, pain is eliminated.
6. Place gauze squares, unfolded, about wound to make sterile field.
7. Open suture; put needle in the needle holder.
8. Grasp one wound margin (side of cut) near the end with tissue forceps. Turn it up to 90° angle. Push needle through, perpendicular to the skin edge (*see* Fig. 18A).
9. Grasp opposite wound margin and repeat step No. 8.
10. Knot the bitter end of the suture to the standing part to close one end of wound.

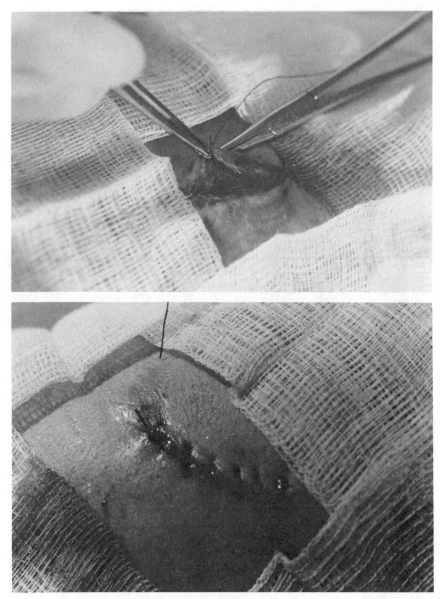

Fig. 18B. Top: Wound suture—first stitch. Note wound margin turned up to a right angle.
18C. Bottom. Completed suture line—suture cut away.

11. Repeat steps No. 8 and No. 9. Fashion a running stitch that closes the whole wound. Keep sides even.
12. Tie a second knot at the other end.
13. Cut the suture free and discard (*see* Fig. 18B).
14. Apply antibiotic ointment to the suture line. Bandage firmly.

The procedure is the same whether you use the materials described or have made substitutes.

FOLLOW-UP CARE OF CLOSED WOUNDS

The procedure is the same for Steri-strips, butterfly or suture-closed wounds.

1. Change outer dressings only if they get wet or very dirty.
2. Remove all dressings in ten days; wound should be healed. Remove closures:
   a. Pull Steri-strips or butterflies off wound edges gently.
   b. Cut sutures at each turn and remove the several fragments. Wipe with antiseptic before you withdraw.
3. Suspect infection at any time after closure if there is:
   a. Increasing pain in wound after 24 hours.
   b. Swelling about wound.
   c. Bulging of wound.
   d. Pus dripping from closure.
   e. Increasing redness and heat about wound.
4. If wound infects:
   a. Remove dressings.
   b. Remove all Steri-strips or sutures.
   c. Spread wound wide open.
   d. Place gauze pads over wound, moisten with salt solution (one tsp. table salt to 1 qt. fresh water). Boil to sterilize.
   e. Keep part at rest and elevated.
5. Suspect wound infection plus sepsis (blood poisoning) if patient has:
   a. Chills and fever (temperature above 101° F.).
   b. Red streaks out from wound.
   c. Swollen tender lymph nodes at groin or axilla.
   d. Points a-e, step No. 3.
6. If wound infection plus blood poisoning (sepsis):
   a. Bunk rest for patient.
   b. Broad spectrum antibiotics: ampicillin 250 mgms (one capsule) at 0800, 1200, 1600, 2000, and 2400 daily.
   c. All procedures under step No. 4.
   d. Use any available antibiotic if no ampicillin. See Chapter VII on antibiotics.
7. Stop wound wet dressing when local infection subsides as shown by:
   a. Less pain and swelling.
   b. Pus stops forming.
   c. Base of wound becomes pink and healthy.
8. Stop systemic antibiotics when temperature is normal for 24 hours and wound shows foregoing changes.
9. After infection subsides, leave wound open to heal in from the bottom. Never close it. Dress as needed with antibiotic ointment; Furacin or Bacitracin and dry gauze.

DISCUSSION—SOFT-PART WOUND HEALING

Soft-part wounds heal much like fractures except that the end product is scar tissue instead of bony callus.

Fine fibrils extruded from blood clot crisscross the wound. Young fibroblast cells creep out along these miniature suspension cables to bridge the gap. They mature into firm scar tissue in from 18 to 21 days.

Infection and/or excessive motion of wound surfaces interrupt proper healing. The wound treatment aims to prevent both.

The outside scrub removes bacteria from the surrounding skin so wound wash and suturing will not carry them into the wound itself. It resembles the skin preparation done before any operation.

Gauze pressed into the wound protects it from splash during the scrub.

The wound washout removes dirt, bacteria and dead tissue that encourage infection.

Careful hemostasis (stopping bleeding) after washout minimizes blood clot in the closed wound. Some clot is needed for healing but an excess promotes infection.

Antibiotic ointment over the wound closure checks bacterial invasion until serum seals the wound shut.

Wound closure shortens healing time by narrowing the valley that healing cells must fill. It also restricts movement of wound edges that might otherwise shear off the delicate developing tissue bridges.

All wounds are contaminated because bacteria are ubiquitous. The bacteria in a fresh wound, however, lie quiet for some hours like newly planted seeds in a field until warmth and moisture incite growth. Usually the body defenses will destroy them before this happens. If not, the bacteria begin to grow and reproduce.

Infection turns the formerly peaceful healing process into a holocaust of battle. Millions of white blood-cell shock troops swarm into the combat along widely dilated arterial pathways. Some of these cells wall in the infection while others gulp down (phagocytose) the deadly bacteria in suicidal attacks. The body count of dead cells and bacteria in the center grows steadily.

Small wonder that trampled nerve ends cause pain, that the part swells and that the heat of violent struggle can be seen and felt through the overlying skin.

Should this first line of defense conquer the infection, there remains a wall of living leucocytes (white blood cells) around the dead cells in the center. This is an abcess and the center is pus.

Pus under pressure can strangle living cells and rally the invader to a renewed attack. Avoid this danger by opening the wound widely to relieve pus pressure. Encourage continued drainage by wet dressings until you see no more pus.

Should the infection overcome this first line of defense it will progress as red streaks in lymph vessels radiating out from the wound. Lymph nodes in armpit or groin will swell and hurt. If it reaches the bloodstream, sepsis (blood poisoning) causes chills, high fever and severe illness.

Systemic antibiotic treatment is necessary to conquer this invasion. The proper use of such drugs is described in Chapter VII.

Leave a wound open once drained, lest you trap some infected material and renew the infection. Such an open wound will heal by second intention. This takes longer and makes more scar than a wound that heals by first intention (i.e., without infection), but it will heal.

Most clean wounds on shipboard should be closed. The less gaposis, the less scar necessary to heal it, and subsequent repair of tendons or nerves will be easier. You will do harm if you attempt to repair deep structures. Close only the skin.

Avulsed wounds, those with the skin torn away, will not close. Approximate wound edges where possible and pack the remaining area with sterile gauze plus antibiotic ointment. Change this when wet or soiled. A wet dressing, warmed by body heat, is an ideal culture media for bacteria.

Badly mangled wounds or those with ground-in dirt (*see* Fig. 19) are best packed open. A good general rule is: if there is any question about closing a wound, pack it open. You will get a bigger scar but will be more likely to have an uninfected wound.

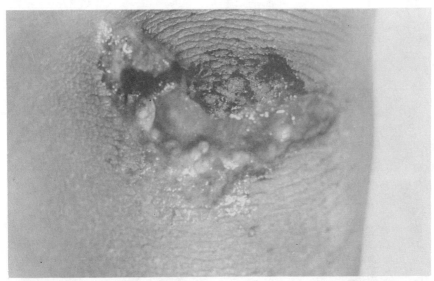

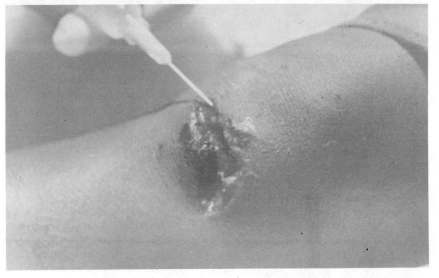

Fig. 19. **Top:** Mangled knee wound—dirt ground into dead tissues. **Bottom:** Injection of local anesthesia before wound scrub-up. **(Continued on next page.)**

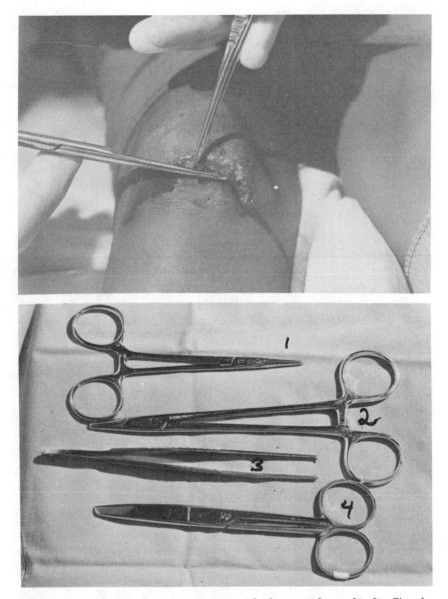

Fig. 19 (continued). Top: Cutting away (scissors) dead tissue and ground-in dirt. Wound to be packed open. **Bottom:** Instrument kit for wound excision and/or suture: 1) hemostat; 2) needle holder; 3) tissue forceps; 4) scissors. Sterilize by boiling 20 minutes.

PUNCTURE WOUNDS

Puncture wounds—deep, narrow holes such as a nail would make—require special treatment. Tetanus (lockjaw) bacilli and gas gangrene bacteria are obligate anerobes. They grow only in the absence of oxygen.

Anerobic conditions develop at the bottom of a deep puncture wound if the top seals over before the bottom heals.

To treat a puncture wound:

1. Inject local anesthesia (1% Xylocaine) into and around such a puncture wound.
2. Core it out.
3. Pack it open with antibiotic ointment on sterile gauze to heal from the bottom up.
4. Additional prevention from tetanus can be assured by immunization of each crew member before the voyage begins. It is effective for one year and can be fully restored by booster injections at yearly intervals for a lifetime. It is no substitute for the proper wound management in Steps 1, 2, and 3.

AMPUTATIONS

You are not likely to be unlucky enough in your cruising to encounter a white whale that mangles a leg of one of your crew. But it is possible you may have to amputate an arm or leg.

Do it only to save life. It is a terrifying experience for both skipper and injured crewman. For the moment, save any extremity—however badly mangled—that has essentially normal color (i.e., not dead white or dusky) and that bleeds from exposed vessels within the area of injury or beyond. Splint it carefully; control pain with Demerol, 75-100 mgms (1-1½ ml or cc) by injection every three to four hours as needed. Prevent infection by giving ampicillin (or other available broad spectrum antibiotics) 250 mgms four times a day until clean healing progresses. This may be a few days, a week, two weeks or even longer. Meanwhile, make every effort to secure help.

If in spite of such care the injured part dies and severe spreading infection begins, the patient suffers chills, high fever (temperature oral to 104° F. or even higher) or perhaps delerium. Pain in the injured extremity becomes progressively worse and worse. The dead tissue turns black or dusky and stinks. Red streaks may climb up the extremity; lymph nodes in the groin or armpit swell up and hurt (*see* Fig. 20).

Gangrene may also develop when bleeding in an extremity thwarts control for several days. Each time you loosen the tourniquet or pressure bandage, vigorous bleeding gushes from the wound. Shortly, the patient bleeds to death or the extremity becomes gangrenous from the continued pressure that cuts off adequate blood flow.

If you have a plentiful supply of ice aboard, you may delay amputation of a gangrenous extremity for some hours or days, perhaps time enough to reach port. Proceed thusly:

1. Demerol 100 mgms by injection if none has been given in the past two hours.
2. Place a tourniquet tightly around the limb two inches above any dead tissue or pus. Once placed, never remove it.
3. Pack the limb below the tourniquet in ice. Keep replenishing the ice.

Within 24 hours the pain lessens, the temperature and pulse drop towards normal (less than 100° F. and less than 100 beats/min.) and the patient is obviously better.

You may safely continue the treatment until the temperature and pulse rise sharply and remain elevated. Do not panic at moderate daily fluctuation of temperature and pulse. The sustained progressive rise of either demands intervention.

Do so when you are sure in your own mind the patient is going to die if you do not.

You are the skipper and will have to be the surgeon. Anyone can amputate a finger or toe. Simply inject 10-15 cc of 1% Xylocaine into the base and cut it off. Use a sterilized pair of tin shears or a heavy knife. Control bleeding with a tourniquet of rubber bands or fine ties. Control pain with Demerol and dress the wound afterwards as often as necessary. Leave wound open.

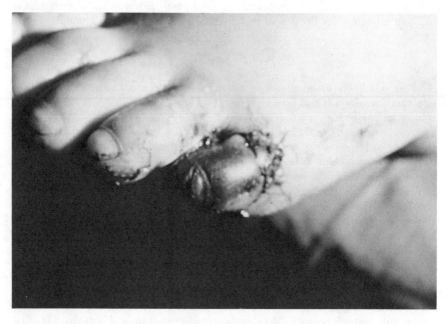

Fig. 20. Gangrenous fifth toe, left. Seven days post suture. Dark area, anesthetic; surrounding foot red, swollen and tender. Amputated—packed open. Healed, 1 week.

If a foot and leg below the knee are involved you can likely amputate successfully. Above the knee you may elect to leave the outcome to fate for amputation at this level is difficult and much more hazardous.

The major danger of the operation is bleeding. It may occur at the time of amputation if the main vessels are not controlled or it may occur up to a week after operation if infection loosens a blood clot in a major vessel.

If you decide you have the courage to go ahead, here is what to do:

1. Get the ship on the steadiest course possible.
2. Select a firm bench or table to which the patient can be lashed and which provides access on all sides.
3. Pick two assistants who do not faint at the sight of blood.
4. Log the date, time and ship's location. Write that in your opinion the patient's life is in danger unless the amputation is carried out. You are not a

doctor but feel competent to remove this offending part and thus save his life. Have the patient sign and both assistants witness this.

Such a consent has no legal standing. However, it is a generally accepted principle of law that what one does in an effort to save a life is usually acceptable.

You will need the following supplies:

1. 100 cc of 1% Xylocaine.
2. A 20 cc sterile syringe with a three-inch needle, size 18 or 20.
3. A sharp knife with at least a three-inch (and preferably a six-inch) blade.
4. Three or four hemostatic forceps.
5. Three dozen sterile gauze squares. If these are not available, tear toweling or sheets into 4 x 4 inch squares and sterilize by boiling for 20 minutes. Then allow to cool and dry before use.
6. Two stout rubber or elastic tourniquets. Mooring slack holders or heavy shock cord are suitable; nylon or Manila line (¼-inch) also.
7. A bucket.
8. Six swedged-on 2-0 silk sutures. If you have no prepared sutures, substitute fishing line, stout packing string, or sail sewing cord and needles (sterilize by boiling 20 minutes).
9. A hacksaw or other type of saw. Sterilize by wiping it several times with antiseptic solution, especially the teeth. A hacksaw is particularly good. Soak the blades in a pan with rubbing alcohol or any other antiseptic for a couple of hours prior to the operation. Have several extra blades.
10. A roll of adhesive tape, 2" x 10 yards.
11. Two Ace bandages, 2-3".
12. A single-action pulley and some means of fastening it to the lower end of the bunk or onto the overhead.
13. Demerol, 50 mgms/ml, 1-ounce bottle.
14. Small (2 cc) hypodermic syringe.
15. Scissors, sterilized.

Preparation of the Patient

1. Give the patient 125 mgms of Demerol plus 10 mgms of Valium by injection one hour before the operation.
2. Shave the entire extremity above the infected area.
3. Scrub the entire leg from groin to toes ten minutes; use fresh water and Phisohex. Make all strokes from clean to dirty area, downward.
4. Lash patient firmly to operating table on a sheet or blanket.
5. Place the bucket immediately below the operative site.
6. Assign second assistant to monitor the tourniquet.
7. Stand on the right side of the patient if it is the right leg and on the left if it is the left leg.
8. Have your first assistant stand directly across from you.
9. Lay your sterile instruments on a clean towel on a handy stand.
10. Scrub your hands for ten minutes with Phisohex and a brush or a soap scrub pad. Rinse with sterile water.

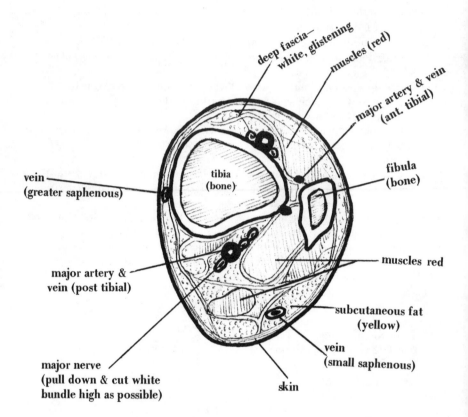

deep fascia—
white, glistening

muscles (red)

major artery & vein
(ant. tibial)

fibula
(bone)

muscles red

subcutaneous fat
(yellow)

vein
(small saphenous)

skin

major nerve
(pull down & cut white
bundle high as possible)

major artery &
vein (post tibial)

vein
(greater saphenous)

tibia
(bone)

Fig. 21. Cross section through left lower leg.

44

Now for the details:

1. Scratch a circle around the leg at the level selected for amputation, two inches above any dead tissue. Use knife tip or a needle.
2. Draw 20 cc of Xylocaine into syringe; inject it into the scratched circle just under the skin. It should bulge the skin all the way around the circle.
3. Refill the syringe and inject around again at a deeper level. Refill the syringe and repeat until you have injected 75-100 cc of Xylocaine and have completely infiltrated tissues from skin to bone in a circle all around the leg.
4. Wait five minutes. Test the anesthesia with a pin below your injection circle. Wait until the leg is numb both on the surface and deep before you begin to operate. The sense of touch may persist but when pain is gone, anesthesia is satisfactory.
5. Second assistant tightens tourniquet firmly about lower thigh. As you operate, if there is any persistent bleeding, tighten the tourniquet until it stops. This is essential; the tourniquet must be tightened until bleeding is controlled. Have a spare tourniquet handy.
6. You have selected a site for amputation at least two inches above any infection or pus or dead tissue.
7. Take your knife, cut clear around the leg through the skin and fat. Follow the scratch. The skin is tough and white; the fat is yellow. Allow a moment for the skin to retract. Fascia glistens white; muscle red below. Then as high as possible towards the retracted skin, cut the muscles all the way around. These will jump and twitch away from your knife but make it as straight as you can. Your first assistant wipes the wound dry of blood with gauze squares so you can see to cut.
8. Continue circular incisions clear around the leg each time until both bones are exposed. There are two bones in the leg: the tibia (large) and the fibula (small).
9. Use the knife to scrape the bone clear for an inch of all muscle attachments and membrane.
10. Inject some local anesthesia (10 cc Xylocaine) into the periosteum, the tough membrane stuck fast to the bone.
11. Unfold a gauze square, wrap it around the divided skin and muscles. Have your second assistant pull up on this hard while your first assistant holds the leg in a handy position.
12. Saw through both bones of the leg. Bones are hard, so brace yourself and the leg. Have extra hacksaw blades available. When both bones are divided, have your assistant drop the amputated extremity into the bucket and chuck it overboard.
13. Find the major arteries as shown in Fig. 21. If you do not locate them easily, let your second assistant release the tourniquet slightly. Watch for the spurting vessels and sew them shut. Use a simple running stitch. If you do not have swedged-on suture materials, use sailmaker's twine and needles from your sail repair kit. Vessels must be sewn; if you simply tie string around them, it may slip off. Tie tightly.
14. When you have secured the major vessels, again release the tourniquet a little to find other bleeding. Sew all the lesser vessels shut or sew muscle bundles together over them.

15. When bleeding is stopped except for a slight oozing, spread a generous amount of Neosporin or Bacitracin ointment over the amputated stump. Do not close the skin.
16. Place Vaseline or plain gauze on top of the Neosporin ointment.
17. Add handfuls of gauze to cover the stump. Wrap firmly with Ace bandages (two or three).
18. Make two adhesive traction strips and stick them to the skin on each side of the leg above the dressing.
19. Move the patient to his bunk. Fasten the traction strips to a line through a block to a weight of about two pounds. This exerts a gentle traction. It is more comfortable and prevents retraction of soft tissues.

FOLLOW-UP CARE OF AMPUTATION

1. Pain control with Demerol 75-100 mgms (1½-2 cc) by injection every three or four hours as necessary for the first few days. Pain will diminish until Emperin and Codeine, ½ gr. by mouth, will suffice.
2. Change dressings as infrequently as possible—only when they become soiled or wet.
3. See instructions for general patient care in Chapters II and III.
4. Give ampicillin 250 mgms every four hours for ten days or until clean healing develops. This will be indicated by less discharge and pink healthy tissues when wound is dressed.
5. **Leave a tourniquet around the lower thigh, loosely at all times.** If bleeding occurs, cinch it up until you can get organized to control it by pressure or by local anesthesia injection and resuture of a bleeding vessel.

Discussion

The gangrenous extremity furnishes excellent soil for deadly bacterial growth while its connections to the living parts above provide excellent channels to spread infection; unchecked it can prove fatal.

The operation described removes this culture media. The wide-open stump allows adequate drainage of any infection that has already reached the lymph vessels and tissue spaces in the living parts above.

It is easier to amputate the leg below, rather than through, the knee. First, it is difficult to cut through the knee joint accurately, and second, the cartilege on the proximal joint surface must be chiseled away—a tedious process. Below-the-knee amputations with salvage of the joint cause considerably less disability than those which sacrifice the joint.

Skin traction applied immediately after operation and held until healing is complete assures adequate soft tissue (muscle and fascia) to provide a good stump—one that can be fitted with an artificial limb.

This procedure can be adapted to amputations of the forearm below the elbow. Follow the same steps, and the anatomy is reasonably similar.

Delayed amputation is really a physiological removal of the limb, i.e., it is externalized completely from the body. This controls infection until it ascends beyond the tourniquet and invades the leg above.

Amputation will have to be done eventually once a permanent tourniquet is set. Often cold will provide enough anesthesia for the amputation with no other local or general anesthetic drug necessary.

SUMMARY

This chapter contains:

1. Case illustrating management of compound fracture of the hand.
2. Management of compound fractures.
    a. Primary definitive.
    b. Follow-up.
3. Discussion of physiology of all fracture healing.
4. Basic principles of managing soft tissue wounds.
    a. Washup of wounds.
    b. Closure by Steri-strip technique.
    c. Closure by sutures.
    d. Follow-up care.
5. Physiology of wound healing.
6. Treatment of special wounds:
    a. Mangled.
    b. Puncture.
7. Amputations.
    a. Indications.
    b. Delaying procedures.
    c. Preparation.
    d. Technique.
    e. Follow-up care.
    f. Physiological principles of amputations.

Chapter IV
BURNS; FLUID ADMINISTRATION

Your trawler, *Nomad*, is rolling along in a heavy following sea, halfway between Turtle Bay and Cabo San Lucas, at a comfortable 10 knots. It's 1200 hours, Tuesday; the galley slave lights off the fires for lunch.

A maverick wave tosses *Nomad* onto her beam ends. There is a scream below and the cook skyrockets up the companionway, hair and clothes ablaze.

First, put out the fire. Don't get burned yourself. Roll him on the deck, wrap him in foul weather gear—anything that's handy.

He sits on the cabin floor; he shivers with fright and pain, an awesome sight; hair and eyebrows singed away; bits of burned clothing hanging on his chest and tummy. He smells like an overdone steak.

1. Control pain and fright.
    a. Cover all burned areas with cool towels, wrung out in fresh water (iced if you have it).
    b. Give him 100 mgms (2 cc) of Demerol by I.M. injection (*see* Fig. 7).
2. Boil three quarts of fresh water in a covered pan for 15 minutes. Let it cool with cover on.
3. Scrub your hands for ten minutes with Phisohex and fresh water.
4. Remove the cold compresses and wash the burns. Use the water you have sterilized, gauze sponges and Phisohex. Clean all areas gently, but thoroughly. By now, the Demerol and cold compresses have dulled his pain.
5. When the burns are cleaned, you must now decide whether he has a serious (i.e., potentially fatal) or a non-serious (painful and annoying) burn.

You determine the severity of any burn by the extent (%) of body surface involved and the depth of injury; the latter expressed in degrees.

The area (%) of the body burned is calculated from the *Rule of Nines* (*see* Fig. 22). The illustration is self-explanatory.

The depth of burn is determined by the appearance of the skin surface.

FIRST DEGREE—redness of skin only (*see* Fig. 23, top).

SECOND DEGREE—blisters (*see* Fig. 23, center).

THIRD AND FOURTH DEGREE—skin surface dead white or brown and insensitive to pinprick (*see* Fig. 23, bottom).

You observe that your patient's scalp (5% of body surface) is blistered—second-degree burn. The front and back of his chest and front of his belly (26% of surface) are involved in second and third degree.

This is a serious burn (potentially lethal); the rule is if 20% or more of body surface is burned to second, third, or fourth degree, the burn is serious.

You may have some difficulty in applying the two determinants. Make a rough estimate of body surface involved from the chart. You may be a bit puzzled about the exact depth in a given area. Do your best. These formulae are designed as a rough guide; as such they are useful. They are about as accurate as an observation of your boat's speed with a chip log and a stopwatch.

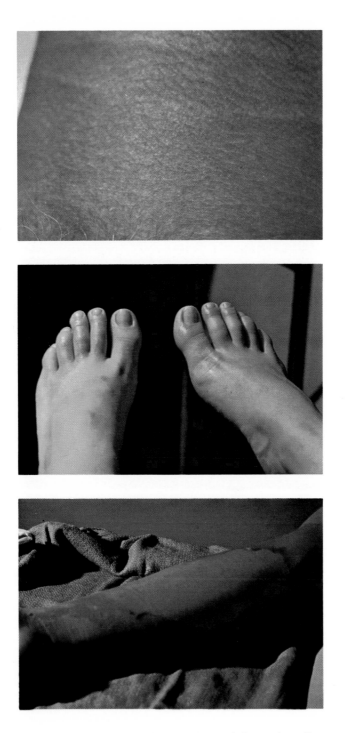

Fig. 23. Top: First-degree burn—redness of skin and swelling.
Center: Second-degree burn—blisters and redness. Bottom:
Third-degree burn—loss of skin—anesthetic to pinprick.

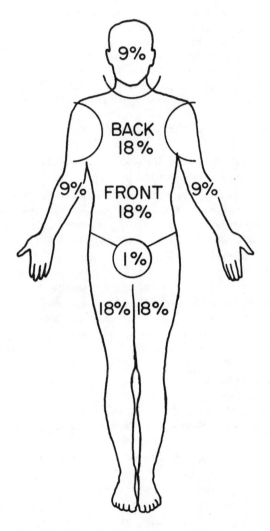

Fig. 22: Rule of nines; percent of body area
burned.

To continue treatment:

6. Reapply the cold compresses for a short time to relieve the pain that was created by the "washup."

7. Remove the cold compresses—apply antibiotic ointment (Furacin) liberally—cover this with sterile gauze patches and then wrap firmly with Ace bandages or Curlex. You may decide to treat the scalp by exposure if you have difficulty fastening a head bandage.

8. Call for help if you have a ship-to-shore phone. Aid may be forthcoming in a few hours or may be delayed for some days.

9. Continue pain control—Demerol (75-100 mgms; 1½–2 cc are average doses and may be repeated at three-hour intervals). The sign of overdosage is increasing drowsiness. In this case, you will discontinue pain injection temporarily.

10. Make several quarts of "salty lemonade" to replace the fluids and minerals lost.

To one quart of water, add one level teaspoonful of table salt, ½ teaspoon of baking soda, and any flavoring available (lemon is best).

11. Urge your patient to drink as much of this as he can without becoming nauseated. Let him drink any fluid that he will, in any quantity (except alcoholic beverages), but urge the salty mixture.

The most serious early complication of a bad burn is burn shock; it may not develop for some hours nor at all, but you must be ready.

Oliguria (diminished urine output), heralds the approach of serious burn shock as clearly as dark clouds on the horizon anticipate a rain squall.

12. As soon as practicable after injury, make the patient empty his bladder. Note the time in the ship's log; throw away the urine.

13. One hour later, have him void again: measure the amount; record in the log at the new time. Discard the urine.

14. Do this every hour for 24 hours.

Let's have a look at the log:

1500—First urine discarded. Unmeasured.

1600—Urine measures 240 cc (8 ounces, one standard measuring cup).

1700—Urine = 120 cc (4 ounces, or ½ standard measuring cup).

1800—Urine = 70 cc (1¼ ounces, or slightly over ¼ cup).

Your patient has voided less than two ounces in the last hour; definite oliguria. Burn shock is on the way.

15. Post a constant watch at his bunk; offer him fluids every ten minutes. Urge him to drink anything he will take. Beer is permissible; no hard liquor.

1900—Urine = 15 cc (½ ounce—barely covers the bottom of the measuring cup).

His personal barometer indicates storms ahead: weakness, rapid pulse, sweating appears, and worst of all he begins to vomit.

Now you will have to give his fluids parenterally. If you don't, his chance for survival is poor.

16. Boil the Kelly bottle and tubing for 10 minutes.

17. Boil three quarts of water in another covered pan for 20 minutes. Turn off the fire and add the proper number of salt tablets (taken from the label on

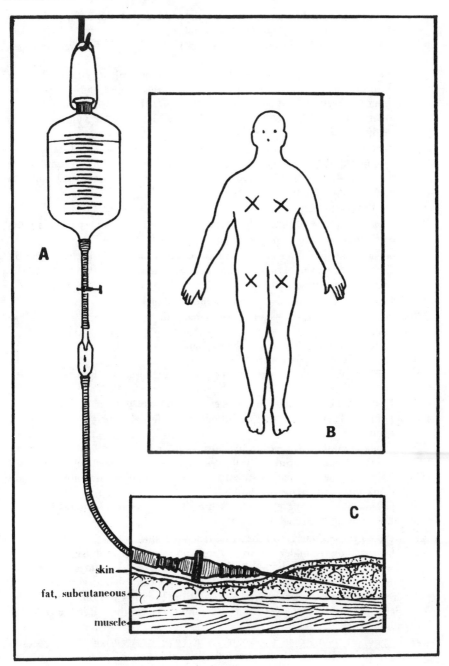

Fig. 24: A) Kelly bottle. B) Sites for fluid injection. C) Position of subcutaneous needle.

the bottle) to make three quarts of normal salt solution. If you have no tablets, add three level teaspoonfuls of table salt.

18. Break out a needle (largest you have—probably No. 18) from prepackaged kit.

19. Hang the Kelly bottle above the patient's bunk; fill it with cooled salt solution; insert the needle into the patient's thigh; open the clamp on the tubing and let the fluid run in under the skin. The leg will swell; it may be moderately painful. It will hurt less if you add 1 cc of 1% Xylocaine (local anesthetic) (see Fig. 24).

20. Insert a Foley catheter inlying into the patient's bladder (see Chap. VI for technique). This enables you to measure hourly urine output more accurately in a very ill patient. Open the catheter clamp each hour to measure urine output.

Continue the log:

2000—Urine = a few drops only from the catheter. Patient pale, clammy, sweating and obtunded; pulse rapid.

21. The subcutaneous fluid swells the right thigh at the site of original injection (one quart of normal salt solution has been given). Move the needle to the left thigh and fill the Kelly bottle again.

2100—Urine = ½ ounce; patient confused and irrational.

2200—Urine = same; patient's condition unchanged.

2300—Urine = ½ ounces.

2400—Urine = 1 ounce. Patient still drowsy and weak.

0100—Urine = ¾ ounce; patient restless.

0200—Urine = 1½ ounces; patient restless, semiconscious, but responds to questions, etc.

0300—Urine = 2½ ounces; patient is less sweaty, more responsive.

0400—Urine = 3 ounces; patient definitely more alert. Has had 3 quarts of salt solution.

0500-Urine = 3 ounces; nausea subsides; drinks some fluid.

0600—Urine = 4 ounces; drinking well; weakness gone and completely alert.

0700—Urine = 8 ounces; patient thirsty and mildly hungry. Give him food and drink. Stop subcutaneous fluids.

Make no mistake—you have saved his life. Without your parenteral fluids he would not have made it through the night.

22. Remove the catheter; stop the subcutaneous fluids.

23. The situation is under control. From now on you will have to change dressings every other day. Give Demerol 100 mgms 45 minutes beforehand; remove the dirty dressings and replace with clean. Should you run out of dressings, leave the last one in place until it becomes too objectionable by sight and smell; then remove it and simply expose the burned area to the air.

24. If you are more than 48 hours from help, start antibiotics by mouth. Ampicillin 250 mgms four times a day or Tetracycline 250 mgms four times a day may be used. If Tetracycline is chosen, avoid the sun; the drug makes one photosensitive.

25. Feed your patient. You have treated a major burn and one which developed the most dreaded early complication—shock. You will turn him over to a physician's care in good condition and have reason to be proud.

Discussion

Burns may vary from a minor annoyance to fatal injuries. Often the severity is immediately obvious but many times it is not.

For example, a third-degree burn of the entire trunk (36% of body surface) is a serious injury. The patient may not appear ill at first.

There is little pain—the deep burn destroys all the nerves to the skin. Pain will develop later when the surrounding intact parts swell up.

It is important, then, to use the rule-of-nines and the depth of burn to determine early after injury what you must expect to treat. It is useful also, in terms of your cruise plans.

Often a burn which looks frightening (blisters of the entire front of the chest) is not serious. It's 9% of body surface, second degree. Local treatment with Furacin and a bandage, something for pain, and in a couple of weeks it will be healed.

First-degree burns (redness only) are rarely important. Sunburn causes most of them. This is painful and annoying but local treatment with cooling compresses together with Emperin and Codeine (½ gr.) will control the pain.

First-degree burns of over 80% of the body surface can become serious and should be carefully watched for development of oliguria. If this occurs, treat the wound as though you were dealing with a deeper burn.

Certain other burns are serious because of the structures involved, even though less than 20% of the body surface is involved.

Burns about the mouth, throat and face may swell and interfere with breathing and swallowing. If an open airway is threatened by such swelling, pass the Resusitube through the mouth and throat before they close.

If swallowing becomes too difficult, administer fluids parenterally.

Third- and fourth-degree burns of an extremity (foot, hand, etc.), although small in size, can cause serious trouble—burned tissues may form the starting place for an overwhelming infection in a few days.

The antibiotics help prevent this. And such a local burn will be less likely to become infected if dried out by air exposure. This is why a burned extremity is best treated by exposure. Bacteria do not grow in dry tissue.

Burns about the rectum or the genitals are also dangerous. The former because it is almost impossible to prevent a burn near the rectum from becoming infected from bowel movements. The latter because, particularly in the male, the penis may swell so that voiding urine is not possible.

Give the patient with a perirectal burn three tablets of Lomotil three times daily to prevent bowel movements. It is possible for the human animal to go for weeks without a bowel movement and this avoids infecting the burn. If a fecal impaction forms, this can be treated later.

If a urogenital burn causes retention, catheterization is necessary.

Treatment of Burns

There are several methods of treating burn wounds. Simple exposure, with various antibiotic ointments and silver nitrate applications to create a scab, are all in use. Or a pressure dressing may be applied and changed as needed.

I consider either method practical for use afloat. Should you not have the necessary bandages, simply expose the burn to air. Place the patient on a clean sheet or blanket; make a tent over him with a spare sail so that he can lie having burns exposed to the air with minimum contact with bedding.

Burn shock, which is the deadliest part of any burn in the first few days, is primarily due to loss of water and salts from the bloodstream. Protein is also lost but there is little one can do about that on shipboard, so we will concentrate on the former.

Oozing from the burns and swelling of the nearby tissues suck fluid from the bloodstream in surprising amounts—four to five quarts each 24 hours in a moderate-sized burn.

The lost fluid slows the blood circulation through the kidney; this produces oliguria which anticipates shock. Hospitals everywhere measure urine output to anticipate the onset of burn shock and to judge the success of fluid therapy.

A modern hospital will study many other parameters of body function when treating a severe burn, but diminished urine output is most reliable.

The other symptoms of burn shock—apprehension, weakness, pallor, nausea, and vomiting—will appear later, but do not wait for these to develop. Replace the fluid; judge your success at this by the urine output; try to keep it above 2 ounces per hour and your patient will survive the initial injury.

This method of giving the parenteral fluid is one of many. It assumes that you will have a Kelly bottle, together with tubing, drip bulb, and some sterile needles in your First-Aid Kit.

These materials can be obtained from any surgical supply house and require less storage space since you will have fresh water aboard.

You may choose, if you have adequate storage space, to buy prepared quart bottles of salt solution. These are sterile, come complete with tubing, needles and printed instructions for their use. For a long cruise (three to six months) half a dozen might be useful. Other conditions (diarrhea, dehydration, heat exhaustion) need them.

If you wish to administer fluids by a more rapid method, intravenously, I advise you to discuss this with your family physician before you start out. The fluids and equipment are similar; difference lies in technique. The subcutaneous method described is learned easily by anyone in five minutes. It is almost foolproof. The insertion of a needle into a vein for intravenous administration is more difficult and hazardous. Perhaps you will have someone aboard familiar with it.

Crush injury, bleeding and major infection, such as peritonitis, may also cause shock.

The symptoms of pallor, rapid pulse, sweating and apprehension or dullness, plus oliguria, will diagnose the condition.

Treat this as you did the burn shock. In addition, if there is high fever (104° F.

or above), give Decadron (adrenal cortical extract) ampules, one by injection every 12 hours for four doses. Give ampicillin, 0.5 gm by injection every 12 hours until temperature remains normal for 24 hours.

You know that dry skin, pounding slow pulse, plus oliguria denote merely simple dehydration and not shock.

SUMMARY
Burns vary from annoying to life-threatening injuries.

1. The extent of any given burn, unless obviously minor, must be determined from the extent of body surface burned and the degree (depth) of injury.

This is important because the critical nature of a given burn may not appear for several hours after injury. Conversely, a burn which appears awesome may be almost harmless.

Treatment:
1. Control the pain and fright.
2. Clean and dress the burn wound.
3. Determine the severity of burn by % area and depth (degree).
4. Anticipate and treat burn shock it if develops.

It is advisable that you discuss with your physician the purchase and use of the various types of sterile fluids and tubing, needles, etc., available before you undertake a long cruise. He will be able to guide you and you will need his prescription to obtain many of the items that have been described.

He may have different ideas of preferable antibiotic ointments and oral antibiotics than these, but he will not change the underlying principles that have been discussed.

Chapter V

HEAT EXHAUSTION AND HEATSTROKE; SEASICKNESS; DEHYDRATION AND DIARRHEA

An April cruise from New York to Barbados puts your cruising ketch, *Restless*, six days out of port heading to warmer weather. All has gone well; you have been reaching all the way and the cold you are leaving behind makes your crew content to stand all watches, even the midwatch, with no complaints.

On the sixth day out, the air temperature rises to 85° F. at 1200 hours and the relative humidity is 85%. Trouble descends upon you like a flight of locusts. Next morning, your port watch captain complains his group has had more than a fair share of night watches and dirty duties.

You review the log with him, point out that this is not entirely true and that it will all even up before you arrive at your destination. The starboard watch captain stands beside you and takes a haughty attitude towards his shipmates' complaints. This does not ease the tension.

You finally straighten it out and the crew goes back to work grumbling. Serenity and joy have left your cruise. Dissension spreads until everyone is griping at everyone else in a way that makes you wish you had never planned a winter cruise.

Thunderheads build up along the horizon. On the eighth day at 1600 hours, a sudden squall demands a sail change. The port watch captain goes forward to douse the Genoa. He hauls the huge sail onto the foredeck as the halyard is paid out; suddenly he collapses.

Others salvage him and the sail. They carry him to his bunk. He lies there gray of face; so weak he can barely fill his lungs with air.

Examine him:

1. Skin wet and clammy.
2. Eyes sunken into their sockets.
3. Pulse at the wrist is hardly perceptible. If you take his blood pressure, you find it low.
4. Oral temperature, 97.8° F., one degree below normal.

You diagnose heat exhaustion. You know now that your whole crew, challenged by heat and humid weather, has suffered a milder form of this disease. It explains the generally rotten dispositions you encountered in the past few days.

But your port watch captain is sick. The others are merely uncomfortable.

1. Wipe him dry with towels.
2. Make two quarts of salty lemonade as described for burns (*see* Chap. IV) and have him sip this.
3. Give him two enteric-coated salt tablets plus a glass of water with each.
4. Keep him warm, covering him with blankets and sheets if necessary.
5. Keep him at rest in his bunk.
6. If he retains the fluids given by mouth, he should be feeling better in an hour or two. Continue the salty lemonade, but now he may have a cup of hot coffee or tea.

7. Give him two enteric-coated salt tablets every four hours until he has had six tablets.
8. If he vomits, stop oral fluids; give him a Compazine suppository or 10 mgms of Compazine by intramuscular injection. Wait half an hour, then start oral salty fluids again.
9. If he vomits after the Compazine, prepare salt solution as described for use in the treatment of burn shock (see Chap. IV). Give him two or three quarts of this subcutaneously as rapidly as he will absorb it. Change injection sites frequently.
10. Avoid non-salt-containing fluids except for the cup or two of coffee or tea.
11. If he does not recover, even though he is retaining salt-containing fluids by mouth or is getting them parenterally, give caffeine and sodium benzoate 7.5 grs. by intramuscular injection.
12. You will judge the success of your treatment by his response. He will feel stronger, his pulse firms up and is slower and he will sweat, but his body will feel warmer to the touch.
13. When he recovers, have him resume his regular duties gradually.

To protect the others, have the galley crew salt all chow heavily and keep enteric-coated salt tablets handy. Anyone who feels weak and excessively sweaty takes a tablet or two with plenty of water.

These measures will prevent severe heat exhaustion and improve dispositions as well.

Another sign of impending heat exhaustion is heat cramps. These occur in the abdominal or leg muscles and come on quite suddenly. They may last a short while or be quite persistent.

HEATSTROKE

Your Barbados cruise has further unpleasant surprises in store. At 1200 hours on the twelfth day out you are trying to rest below decks away from the 100° F. heat and the hot sunlight. There is a sudden yell for you from topside.

You dash up the ladder just in time to see the helmsman slump forward and let the wheel spin. A watch mate grabs it and brings you back on course.

"What's the matter?" you ask the fallen shipmate.

"I'm hot and dizzy and my head is pounding like the devil," he says. He slithers onto the cockpit floor and passes out.

Examination shows:

1. He is unconscious.
2. Skin is dry.
3. No sweating.
4. Forehead is hot to your touch and livid red in color.
5. Pulse is full and bounding.

You recognize heatstroke. Treatment is urgent.

1. Get him below, out of the sun, at once.
2. Log his rectal temperature; if below 103° F., cool him gradually with alcohol or cool water sponges. If his temperature is over 103° F. (and likely

it will be), heroic measures are necessary. Strip him naked and sluice him down with buckets of cold or ice water.

3. Log successive rectal temperatures every 30 minutes; when one drops below 102° F., stop the cooling measures.
4. Dry him off and put him in his bunk with light covering.
5. If he becomes irrational, delirious or hyperactive, give Valium 10 mgms by injection.
6. As he begins to recover, give him food and non-alcoholic fluid as he wishes.
7. Give Emperin and Codeine ½ gr. or aspirin 10 grs. every 3—4 hours as necessary for headache.
8. When his headache subsides and his temperature has been normal for 24 hours, allow him to resume his normal activities.
9. Put him on night watches for the rest of the cruise and keep him below deck as cool as possible and out of the sun in the daytime.

Discussion

Heat exhaustion and heatstroke represent failures in the physiological mechanisms that dissipate heat. Each condition deranges different body defenses and produces a different, though related, group of symptoms.

The body needs water for all its functions including heat loss. Daily requirements under ordinary conditions are:

1. 1000 cc to moisten air breathed.
2. 500 cc for minimal or insensible perspiration (perspiration that is so slight as to pass unnoticed, but is always present).
3. 1000 cc for urine excretion.

This water is obtained from:

1. Liquids and semisolid foods (lean cooked meat, for example, is 60-70% water).
2. Oxygenation (burning) carbohydrate, protein and fat in body metabolism.
   100 gms fat burned = 107 gms water.
   100 gms carbohydrate burned = 55 gms water.
   100 gms protein burned = 41 gms water.

The body also requires certain minerals; the chief one for purposes of this discussion is sodium chloride or ordinary table salt.

The average 150-lb. man on the usual diet will excrete at least 2.5 gms of sodium chloride in the urine and sweat daily. This amount has to be replaced since the body cannot manufacture it.

Much greater amounts of salt and water may be lost with exercise during warm humid weather. A football player, for instance, may lose 1400-1500 cc of water and 3-5 gms of salt in one hour's play on a warm September day.

Water replacement alone will not suffice. Salt must also be taken. The body is a chemical machine and homeostatic mechanisms of infinite complexity operate continuously to maintain the concentration of electrolytes (in this case, salt) constant since within reasonable limits it is the concentration of electrolytes rather than the absolute amount present that determines chemical activity. If total body salt content is low, the kidneys will excrete body water to restore normal concentration. If water is given by mouth without salt when the salt stores of the body are depleted, the water will be excreted at once.

The salt and water carry heat via the bloodstream from the internal cells of the body where it is manufactured to the lungs and skin surface where it can be lost. It is similar to the transport of heat in your automobile engine from the block to the radiator.

When salt and water are lost through excessive perspiration due to work in a hot and humid atmosphere, the total volume of body fluids is diminished. If plain water is drunk, it is not retained. Eventually such fluid losses reduce the volume of blood circulating until a shock-like state develops, somewhat similar to that following a severe burn. This shock state lowers body metabolism and body temperature since oxygen transport to the tissue is diminished. Hence the person suffering from heat exhaustion feels weak, his body is cold and clammy, his temperature subnormal and his blood pressure low.

Treatment provides salt and fluid to restore the circulating volume.

Heatstroke, a much more dangerous condition, results when the external environment prevents heat loss from the lungs and skin. Extremely high air temperature or moderately high, plus excessive humidity, creates this climate. The temperature of the blood rises. This in turn knocks out the sensitive heat control center at the base of the brain. The blood vessels to the skin close down (vasoconstrict), sweating stops, and so does heat loss.

The person with heatstroke, as you noted, was hot and did not sweat. Delerium, convulsions, coma and death proceed in rapid order with true heatstroke.

The treatment is external body cooling. If the temperature is moderately elevated, this may be gradual. If the temperature is above 103° F., it must be rapid and heroic. Valium, 5-10 mgms by injection, helps control convulsions or delerium.

The thoughtful skipper protects his crew from heatstroke and heat exhaustion by anticipation. His cruise will be more enjoyable too, because such measures prevent development of a minor degree of heat exhaustion that causes general grouchiness.

External temperatures of 80° F., with a relative humidity of 50% or over sounds the alert. A wet and dry bulb thermometer records humidity. It is a must for hot weather or tropical cruising. The relative humidity is important because the more saturated the air with water vapor, the less evaporation and cooling occurs from the body surface. To further our analogy, it would be like submerging the car radiator in a steam bath and expecting it to lose heat readily.

The first few days of exposure to this type of atmosphere are the most dangerous.

After a short period of time, the body acclimatizes to increases of heat and humidity by:

1. Dilation of the blood vessels in the skin with greater surface radiation heat loss.
2. Increased perspiration with low salt content. More evaporation cooling, and saves body salt stores.
3. Increasing total body fluid volume to implement these mechanisms.
4. Decreasing excretion of salt in the urine.

Athletic trainers and coaches know acclimatation takes from five to fifteen days. Therefore, during first warm weeks of the football season, workouts are kept at a minimum, extra water and salt are made available, and light clothing is worn. In addition, practice sessions are planned to some degree according to daily variations of temperature and humidity.

When you first reach a subtropic climate with a crew that is unacclimatized, you should:

1. Have everyone wear light protective clothing, headgear and sunglasses that protect from the sun.
2. Shorten daytime watch hours; two on and two off, instead of four on and four off, during the heat of the day.
3. Have frequent cooling on deck. Sluice members of the watch with a bucket of sea water from time to time, or rig a shower with a grill placed in the bottom of a sea anchor. This frequent cooling is similar to spot coolers on merchant and naval ships. In the engine rooms, huge blowers blast cool air and from time to time, members of the engine-room gang stand under one. It enables them to tolerate an otherwise unbearble temperature and humidity.
4. Diet should provide adequate fluids, plenty of carbohydrates; protein foods should be avoided, since their ingestion is followed by increased body heat.
5. Provide enteric-coated salt tablets. They dissolve only in the small intestine, are absorbed more rapidly, and do not cause vomiting with high salt concentration in the stomach.

SEASICKNESS

A wise skipper leaves the persistently seasick ashore when he embarks on a long ocean race or cruise. It is hard to do for many reasons, not the least of which is that such folk will often hide this weakness in the hope of being asked to go along. But it must be done with perception and thoroughness.

Drugs will control seasickness but too often substitute drowsiness. If you depend on them for a long haul, you may wind up coddling a sleepy slob while all hands double up to stand his watches.

Many sailormen suffer mild seasickness at the start of a voyage but acquire sea legs in a day or two. These make good crewmen; the steadily seasick do not.

Extreme weather conditions (slatting, windless for several hours in a huge ground swell) may induce the hardiest sailor to lose his lunch. If vomiting continues, he will lose his vigor and interest in the cruise as well.

Compazine, by suppository or 10 mgms by injection, will usually control vomiting. If the sufferer is unable to retain salt and water after this drug, prepare and give him salt solution parenterally as described for burn shock in Chapter IV.

DIARRHEA

Protracted diarrhea may lead to dehydration with marked weakness. Oral replacement with salty lemonade (see Chap. IV) will restore vigor.

Concurrent vomiting that cannot be controlled by Compazine demands administration of parenteral salt solution (see Chap. IV).

Two Lomotil tablets three times a day will control diarrhea in the absence of vomiting.

Measuring and recording urine output is the best method of determining if fluid replacement, whether by mouth, under the skin or into the vein, is successful. A urine output of 900 cc or more per 24 hours indicates that treatment is correcting dehydration.

SUMMARY

Crew exposure to air temperature of 80° F. or higher, with relative humidity of 50% or greater, poses the threat of heat exhaustion and heatstroke.

Greatest danger is upon first exposure, since the body can acclimatize to this strain if given proper aid over the first week of exposure.

Additional salt and water, proper clothing, frequent cooling and shorter daytime watches will help avoid serious symptons during this period of adjustment. These measures should be continued during the entire period of exposure.

Heat exhaustion is a shock-like state characterized by weakness, coldness, low body temperature and low urine output. It develops when excess salt and water are lost from the body and not replaced.

Treatment of heat exhaustion consists of replacement of salt and water.

Heatstroke, more dangerous but fortunately more rare, occurs when the external environment prevents normal loss of heat. Temperature of the blood rises. Headache, elevated blood pressure, dry skin, delerium, coma and death may develop.

Treat heatstroke by external cooling of the body; rapidly if the temperature is high and the patient unconscious. Give Valium 10 mgms by injection to control delerium and/or convulsions.

Chronic, persistent seasickness is eliminated by careful selection of the crew.

Acute seasickness under extreme weather conditions is controlled by anti-emetic drugs (Compazine) and oral or parenteral fluids containing salt.

Diarrhea may also produce fluid and electrolyte loss and require replacement, in addition to control of excessive bowel movements.

Chapter VI

ABDOMINAL PAIN AND GENITOURINARY
EMERGENCIES

One day as you cruise 1,000 miles from the nearest port, you note one of your crew skips morning chow. File it in the back of your mind for attention later on in the day.

He passes a second meal. Ask him why he is not eating.

"Got a bellyache," he says, "but it isn't bad."

1. Do not accept this evaluation. Take him someplace remote from the wisecracks of the rest of the crew and ask:
    a. Did pain or nausea start first?
    b. Where is the pain? How bad is it, really?
    c. Has it changed its location since it began?
    d. Do you feel like vomiting?
    e. Is it getting worse or better?
    f. Does walking make your stomach hurt? If so, where?
    g. Have you ever had a pain like it before?
2. Have him lie flat on his back with his whole belly exposed.

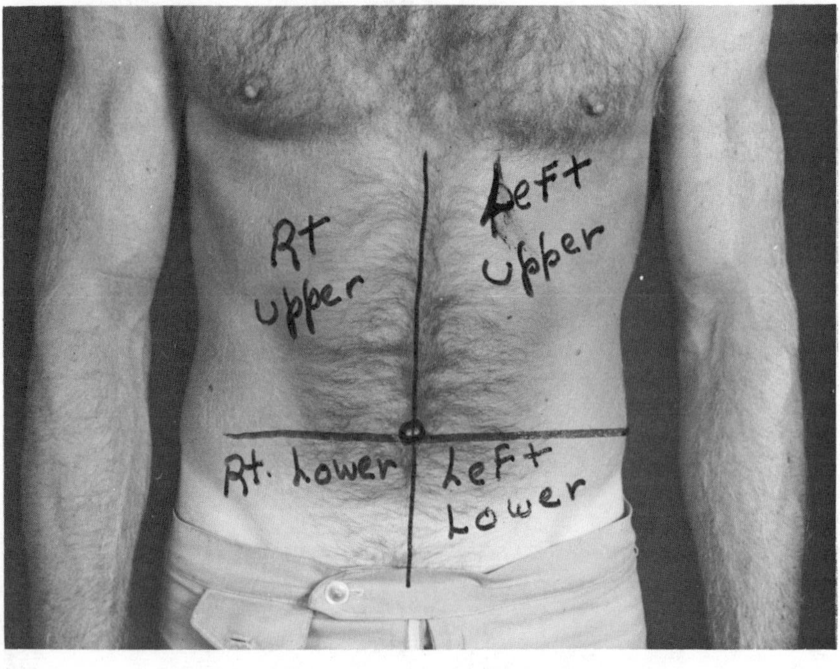

Fig. 25. Abdominal examination—the four quadrants.

3. Rub your hands to warm them; gently, with palms flat, press each of four abdominal quadrants, right and left upper and lower. Note any tender areas (*see* Fig. 25).
4. Take his temperature.
5. Log the above findings in detail.
6. Have him take an enema, prepackaged or homemade (*see* Fig. 26).

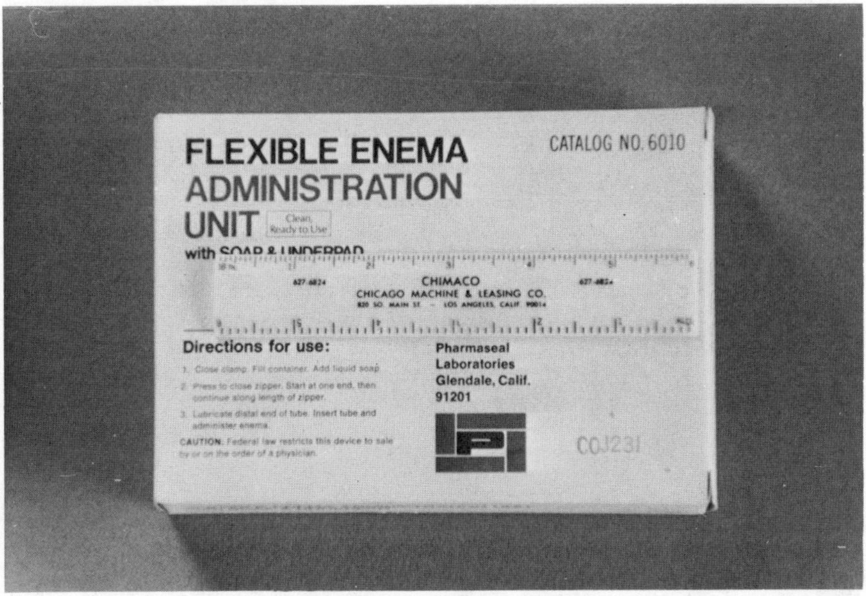

Fig. 26. Prepackaged enema kit.

If his pain persists 12 hours following the enema:

1. Get him off his feet.
2. Allow only water, tea or coffee without cream or sugar by mouth.
3. Repeat your examination now and every six hours (history, oral temperature, belly palpation). Log all observations.
4. Continue above measures until appetite returns, temperature becomes normal, pain stops and belly is not tender at all. Then he may get up and go to duty.

If, on the other hand, a subsequent six-hour examination discovers:

1. Persistent nausea or vomiting.
2. Worse pain in belly.
3. Pain shifts to right lower abdomen and stays there (*see* Fig. 27).
4. Rebound tenderness, lower right abdomen. (This is a sharp stab of pain when firm hand pressure on belly is suddenly released).
5. Fever, temperature 99° or higher.
6. Walking or jumping on right foot causes pain in right lower abdomen.

If 1–6 inclusive are present, suspect acute appendicitis—probably unruptured as yet.

If 1, 2 and 5 are present but tenderness is in the upper belly, acute cholecystitis, duodenal ulcer or some other disease is present (*see* Fig. 27).

The following treatment is effective for painful abdominal disease at this stage, whatever the underlying etiology.

Give:

1. Clear liquids only by mouth (water, tea; no milk or sugar).

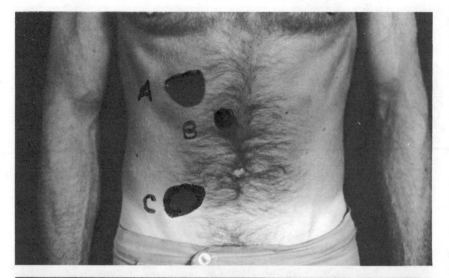

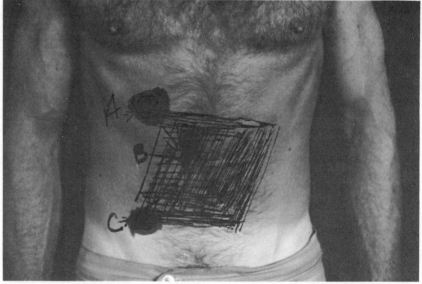

Fig. 27. Top: Abdominal tenderness. A) Acute cholecystitis. B) Duodenal ulcer—simple. C) Acute appendicitis. **Fig. 28. Bottom:** Spread of tenderness and spasm—originating at C) from ruptured appendix; B) from perforated ulcer; A) from ruptured gallbladder (rare). This is peritonitis.

2. Demerol, 75-100 mgms (1½-2 cc) by injection every 3–4 hours as needed to control pain.
3. Keep patient in his bunk except to use the head.
4. Give ampicillin 250 mgms by mouth at 0800, 1400, 2000, and 0200 hours daily. Use other antibiotics if no ampicillin is available. Broad spectrum antibiotics are preferred.

The patient may improve (less pain and tenderness in belly, nausea subsides, temperature becomes normal) in 24–36 hours and he will be well in a few days with such treatment.

When you are sure all pain, abdominal tenderness and fever are gone, continue treatment one day longer. Then feed him and put him back to duty.

If, instead, he gets worse (more pain, vomiting, abdominal distension, more tenderness and rebound tenderness, temperature 101-103° F., pulse 100/min or more), the infection is spreading from its original focus to invade the peritoneal cavity. This is peritonitis (see Fig. 28).

Maximum tenderness in right lower abdomen suggests a ruptured appendix; tenderness and muscle spasm all over the abdomen suggests a perforated ulcer; local signs in right upper abdomen point to acute cholecystitis.

You treat peritonitis from whatever source as follows:

1. Give ampicillin by intramuscular injection, 0.5 gm every 12 hours.
2. Give 1500 cc salt solution by subcutaneous injection (see Chap. IV).
3. Measure and record during first 24 hours of treatment: (measuring cup=8 ounces=240 cc. Coffee cup, also 8 ounces).
   a. Subcutaneous fluid actually given.
   b. Water drunk.
   c. Urine output.
   d. Oral loss by vomiting or nasogastric tube suction (see Step No. 7).

You should have a fluid balance log like this:

Intake

Subcutaneous: salt solution	1300 cc	actually absorbed by patient.
Sips of water by mouth	1000 cc	
Total intake fluid/24 hours	2300 cc	

Output

Urine	800 cc
Vomited	100 cc
Total output fluid/24 hours	900 cc

4. To compute fluid needs for next (second) 24 hours:

Take basic daily requirement =	1500 cc	salt solution
Add left over from 1st day (unable to give it all) =	300 cc	
	1800 cc	
Subtract water drunk =	-1000 cc	
	800 cc	

Give in second 24 hours by subcutaneous injection: 800 cc salt solution.

    5. Compute fluid requirement each 24 hours as shown above. Fifteen hundred cc daily basic salt solution required each 24 hours, plus amount equal to loss by vomiting or stomach suction (*see* Step No. 7), minus water drunk preceding 24 hours.

    6. If urine output drops below 500 cc during any 24-hour period, raise basic daily salt solution from 1500 cc to 2000 cc each 24 hours by subcutaneous injection.

    7. Should the patient vomit repeatedly, pass a nasogastric tube. This rests the bowel. To pass a nasogastric tube:

    a. Assemble stomach tube, lubricant, bulb syringe.

    b. Sit patient upright in his bunk.

    c. Lubricate tip of nasogastric tube (Vaseline, salad oil, etc.).

    d. Give patient a cup of water to hold in his right hand.

    e. Insert the tip of tube into one nostril; point it down towards the floor of the nose cavity.

    f. Push it steadily into his nose.

    g. When the tube hits back of patient's throat, have him swallow water from the cup in his hand.

    h. Keep pushing the tube; have him keep swallowing. You will feel the tube hang up a bit at the Cardio-esophageal junction (where the gullet or esophagus joins the stomach). Then it will pop into the stomach. The mark on the tube shows when it is in the stomach.

    i. Tape tube to forehead. Check the position in stomach by suction on the tube with the bulb syringe. You should get back some bile, stained or whitish acid-smelling stomach fluid.

Passing the stomach tube is often not this easy. After a swallow of water, the patient will retch, the tube will come flying out of his mouth along with a quart or so of vomit. Never mind; you have emptied the stomach—not as neatly as you might wish, but effectively. Rest a moment; pull tube from his nose and start over. When you finally get it in place, vomiting will stop.

If the patient takes a few deep breaths and makes vigorous efforts at swallowing, you will usually get the tube into the stomach.

    j. Keep the stomach empty by suction with the bulb syringe or hang the end of the nasogastric tube into a basin on deck. Siphonage will keep emptying stomach secretion.

If the tube drains correctly, the stomach will be empty and then the patient will not vomit. If tube plugs up, clear it by injection of one ounce of water with bulb syringe. It may improve drainage to untape tube from forehead and move it up or down a few inches.

    8. If temperature recedes, pain lessens, vomiting subsides and abdominal tenderness goes away, the patient is getting better. Remove the stomach tube when nausea subsides. Stop the parenteral salt solution when he can drink enough to keep urine output over 500 cc/24 hours.

Feed him whatever he will eat when he gets hungry. Stop antibiotic injections when oral temperature has been normal for 24 hours. Read Chapter VII, *The Use of Antibiotics.*

9. Should he get worse rather than better (higher fever, pain more severe, persistent nausea, tenderness spreading over the abdomen), continue treatment. This will keep him alive until you reach port.

Discussion—Abdominal Pain

Common causes of abdominal pain are dietary indiscretion, constipation and gastroenteritis (commonly called intestinal flu).

More serious, though fortunately less common causes, are appendicitis, acute cholecystitis, gallbladder infection and duodenal ulcer disease.

Life afloat encourages constipation. Irregular hours, inactivity, dehydration and limited head facilities discourage crews from daily bowel movements, particularly the shy guys.

On one transpacific sailboat race, we kept a paper tacked up in the head. Each sailor checked off a daily passage. If he skipped two days, he ate an extra ration of prunes or took a cathartic. It worked well.

Constipation causes bellyaches so often that the first step in diagnosis of abdominal pain is to give the patient an enema. Relief frequently follows.

Gastroenteritis, or "intestinal flu," is usually caused by a virus and shows itself by nausea and diarrhea. Treatment is rest and Lomotil to control the fluid loss from frequent bowel movements. Codeine will also slow diarrhea if you lack Lomotil.

A male previously well starts an attack of acute appendicitis with a moderate pain located somewhat vaguely throughout the upper abdomen. Nausea follows shortly. It is axiomatic that unless pain precedes nausea, appendicitis is not the trouble. In a few hours, or perhaps a day or two, the pain migrates to the right lower abdomen and settles there. It becomes increasingly severe and eventually tenderness (which differs from the pain in that you must touch the patient to determine it) develops over the site of the appendix. It is located in the right lower abdomen (see Fig. 27).

Appendicitis starts as a minute abscess in the appendiceal wall. Too small to hurt at first, it nevertheless flashes a message back along the nerves in the bowel wall to stop further progress of all food and fluid from above.

This clamps down the pylorus muscle at the outlet of the stomach. Spasm of this muscle causes the early pain in the upper abdomen during the attack of acute appendicitis.

The abscess in the appendix enlarges and begins to hurt locally; the pain moves down to the right lower quadrant of the abdomen and the overlying belly wall becomes sensitive to touch.

The infection at this point is still localized to the appendix. The disease is not serious yet. The potential for harm is great.

It is now, while infection is still limited to the appendix, that rest, antibiotics and control of pain with Demerol offer the best chance of curing the disease. The infection subsides; the patient gradually recovers. This is the importance of early attention to bellyache.

Should the abscess enlarge to burst the appendiceal wall, the infection spreads throughout the abdominal cavity. This is peritonitis (see Fig. 28).

Rupture of the appendix is frequently followed by sudden relief of pain. For an hour or two, the patient feels much better. Shortly, however, temperature rises, nausea and vomiting recur, pain returns and tenderness spreads outward in all directions from the original site in the right lower abdomen. The abdominal muscles harden into spasm to protect the painful guts beneath.

Be sure when treating suspected acute appendicitis that sudden relief of symptoms is permanent before you stop treatment.

Should the appendix rupture, supportive treatment (rest, parenteral fluids and antibiotics, bowel rest and pain control), offers the body's natural defenses a chance to control peritonitis. Infected bowel loops secrete an adhesive exudate and stick together to localize or "wall off" the infection into an abscess. When you reach port, a surgeon can drain this.

The foregoing describes the classic onset and course of acute appendicitis. Unfortunately, this disease is atypical as often as classic. Experienced surgeons often puzzle over the diagnosis.

To reiterate:

The skipper's approach to the threat of acute appendicitis is to start treatment when:

1. A previously healthy male* gets a bellyache.
2. The bellyache lasts 12 hours or longer.
3. An enema does not stop the bellyache promptly.

The treatment outlined aims to prevent acute appendicitis from progressing to a ruptured appendix, although this is not always possible. It also can sustain life if this catastrophe occurs.

If diagnosis is incorrect, the treatment outlined will do no harm.

Certain individuals entering into high office and a few adventurers have undergone elective surgical removal of a normal appendix prior to setting out upon their various journeys.

This is possible, reasonably safe and is a matter to be settled by each individual in discussion with his family physician.

ACUTE CHOLECYSTITIS–GALLBLADDER INFECTION

This disease differs from acute appendicitis in seagoing qualities.

1. It is uncommon in men—actually rare below the age of 35 years. A surgical axiom states that acute cholecystitis occurs typically in fair, fat, 40-year-old flatulent females.
2. It is a recurrent disease. Sufferers have usually had prior attacks and know what to do about them.
3. It is more dramatic than acute appendicitis. The pain can send the bravest rolling to the deck in agony. The victim's skin and eyeballs may turn bright yellow. He may void orange-colored urine.
4. It is a less dangerous disease than acute appendicitis in spite of the melodrama of symptoms. The infected gallbladder rarely ruptures to cause peritonitis.

---

*Note: This is not male chauvinism; females have frequent pain in lower right belly due to ovarian function and so are less suspect of appendicitis from bellyache.

5. The pain and soreness start in the upper abdomen and remain there. There is no definite sequence of pain followed by nausea, as in acute appendicitis. Vomiting, however, is common.

Treatment is designed to maintain fluids, provide antibiotics and relieve pain.

Treat suspected acute cholecystitis exactly as you do suspected acute appendicitis with the addition of atropine 1/150 grs. by injection every six hours for the first 48 hours.

Discussion—Acute Cholecystitis—Gallbladder Infection

The gallbladder recycles water and certain important chemicals. It also helps digest fatty foods. It is a useful but not essential organ.

Bile formed in the liver consists mainly of bilirubin (a pigment derived from breakdown of red blood hemoglobin), bile salts, calcium and cholesterol.

The gallbladder receives this mixture and withdraws water plus bile salts into the blood for reuse.

When fats are eaten, the gallbladder contracts and splashes a generous dollop of concentrated bile onto them as they emerge from the stomach into the duodenum. This bile emulsifies fat for digestion. Should the gallbladder be removed surgically, the bile duct system takes over the concentrating function.

Bile in the gallbladder, for reasons presently obscure, sometimes precipitates stones of calcium, bilirubin and cholesterol, substances normally held in solution. Such stones may move to block the narrow cystic or common ducts.

In either instance, the blocked bile builds back pressure that overdistends the gallbladder.

The gallbladder contracts violently to overcome the obstruction caused by the stone plugging the duct. It is violent contraction against obstruction that causes gallbladder colic which hurts as much as any pain humans suffer.

If the obstruction is in the common duct, bile backs up through the liver into the bloodstream. The patient turns yellow (jaundice), and voids orange-colored urine (bilirubinemia).

Unless the obstructing stone falls back into the gallbladder or is pushed forward through the common duct, the disease persists until a surgeon removes the stone. He usually removes the diseased gallbladder, as well, to prevent formation of future stones.

However, the sturdy gallbladder wall sustains back pressure for long periods and perforation with peritonitis due to bile is rare. Usually the stone obstructs only the cystic duct and falls back into the gallbladder with complete relief after a few days.

Atropine relaxes the muscle in the gallbladder wall.

Acute cholecystitis tends to recover spontaneously rather than rupture and produce the serious complications that follow a ruptured appendix.

Recovery from an attack of gallstone disease is, however, usually only temporary because stones are present and may obstruct again at any time.

It is desirable for anyone with proven gallstone disease to have it surgically corrected before cruising long distances.

DUODENAL ULCER

The pain of duodenal ulcer is located in the right upper quadrant of the abdomen and develops when the stomach is empty.

A small amount of bland food, or antacid, will bring a temporary relief for pain but it will recur after a varying interval.

Diagnosis of duodenal ulcer:

1. Right upper abdominal pain when stomach is empty.
2. Milk, bland foods or antacids give temporary relief of the pain.
3. There will be a tender spot to the right and a bit above the belly button (*see* Fig. 27).
4. The patient may have a history of ulcer disease.

Treatment of duodenal ulcer:

1. Bland diet; any type of meat cooked any way but fried (except bacon, pork or sausage).
2. Any cooked vegetables except onions or cabbage.
3. Any canned or cooked fruits.
4. Any starches; potatoes (except fried), rice, tapioca.
5. No alcoholic beverages.
6. No smoking.

Program:

1. 0800 — Breakfast:
   Eggs (any style but fried); powdered eggs good. Milk, powdered or canned. Cereal, tea, white bread, oatmeal, butter. No coffee.
2. 1000 hours - Snack:
   Glass of powdered milk or crackers, cereal, or bread and two ounces of Gelusil or other antacid.
3. 1200 hours — Lunch:
   Sandwiches or macaroni and cheese, or rice, canned meats (except highly spiced).
4. 1600 hours — Repeat snack.
5. 1800 hours — Supper:

Canned, broiled or boiled meat, canned or any cooked fruit. Any potatoes, boiled, broiled *(not fried)* rice pasta, cooked vegetable (except onions).

Discussion—Duodenal Ulcer

A healthy stomach secretes just enough hydrochloric acid to digest food actually present or anticipated by sight and smell of a meal.

The stomach grinds the food, mixes it with acid and other enzymes and passes this acid chyme through the pylorus into the duodenum.

The duodenal content (pancreatic and intestinal juices plus bile) is alkaline and promptly neutralizes the incoming acid chyme. This protects the duodenal mucosa which is resistant to alkali but not to acid.

The stomach of a duodenal ulcer sufferer secretes acid continually whether or not food is present in the stomach. This excess acid, unmixed with food, squirts through the pylorus, strikes the duodenal wall and erodes the lining; this forms a duodenal ulcer. It is usually about ½-¾" in diameter.

The cause of acid hypersecretion is a mystery, although stress, nervous influences and personality types appear to play some part.

The ulcer, once formed, hurts when bathed in acid. Food or antacids absorb the acid and give temporary relief. A bleeding ulcer filled with blood hurts very little for the same reason.

Treatment simply keeps bland food and/or antacid constantly in the stomach to soak up the acid and let the ulcer heal.

Most duodenal ulcers so treated heal.

If untreated, the ulcer may erode an artery and bleed, or even perforate the muscle coats of the duodenal wall.

ACUTE PERFORATION OF DUODENAL ULCER

A male with past history of recurrent bellyache or diagnosed duodenal ulcer awakes at 0400 hours groaning with pain. It doubles him up; he feels cut in two through his upper belly.

The pain gradually spreads (an hour to two or three) over the entire abdomen. He retches, but raises no vomit (*see* Fig. 28).

Examine him:

1. Apprehensive, sweating, pale and in severe pain.
2. Pulse 100 beats/min. or faster.
3. The abdomen is rigid, boardlike; if thumped, it sounds and feels like a wooden table.
4. Temperature (oral) subnormal and gradual elevation over next 12 hours.

Treatment for suspected perforated ulcer:

1. Absolutely nothing by mouth.
2. Demerol 75-100 mgms (1½-2 cc) by injection soon and every four hours as necessary for pain.
3. Pass nasogastric tube, continuous siphon or bulb suction to keep stomach empty.
4. Log fluid intake and output as for acute appendicitis.
5. Supply daily subcutaneous fluids—as for appendicitis acute. Give ampicillin 1.0 gm by intramuscular injection every 12 hours.
6. If patient has difficulty voiding, pass catheter and leave inlying. This probably will not be necessary.
7. Keep patient in his bunk.

Follow-up care—perforated ulcers 5-10 days or even longer:

1. Keep patient bunk-fast, control pain, supply parenteral fluids and antibiotics, until:
   a. Nausea and pain subside.
   b. Oral temperature is normal.
   c. Abdominal tenderness and rigidity relent.
2. Stop antibiotics when oral temperature is normal for 24 hours.
3. When abdominal pain and nausea completely subside, clamp the stomach

tube shut. If patient does not vomit in six hours, remove the tube. If he does vomit before this time, reopen the tube and continue the siphonage and drainage a bit longer. After the tube is removed, start sips of water by mouth, gradually increasing to full bland diet, and resume program described for treatment of uncomplicated ulcer.

4. Allow patient out of his bunk when all symptoms subside, when he is eating bland diet and feels strong. It will be some time before he is able to resume any duties aboard ship.

Discussion of Perforated Duodenal Ulcer

After perforation, a hole in the duodenal wall replaces the ulcer. This defect allows the acid and alkaline secretions of the gut, plus ingested food and fluids, to leak into the peritoneal cavity.

These digestive enzymes burn the peritoneal surfaces and produce a chemical peritonitis. The systemic effect on circulation and regular body metabolism is similar to that produced by heat burn on the body surfaces. Untreated, such peritonitis is a distinct threat to life.

The peritoneal cavity can defend itself from the single spill at the time of perforation provided that it stops promptly.

Treatment aims to stop it. Nothing is taken by mouth and the nasogastric tube sucks out indigenous secretions as fast as they form.

The great omentum, a fold of peritoneum hung from the stomach, then swings over the perforation in the duodenum. It secretes a sticky exudate similar to that made by inflamed bowel loops after a ruptured appendix. In a few days this will seal off the hole.

Meanwhile, you must sustain life with parenteral fluids and prevent infection with antibiotics.

BLEEDING DUODENAL ULCER

A 26-year-old sailor comes from the head, puzzled. He has just had a large, black liquid bowel movement. "It looks gummy and black like tar," he says, "and I feel weak and dizzy."

1. Ask him:
   a. "Have you ever had an ulcer before?"
      He says, "Two years ago I had stomach pain, X-rays proved negative for ulcer. My doctor gave me antacids and a bland diet and the pain stopped."
   b. "Have you had any pain in your stomach lately?"
      "No, I haven't."
   c. "Do you feel like vomiting?"
      "Yes, a little bit."
2. Examine him:
   a. He is pale and frightened looking (even under a good suntan).
   b. Pulse 90-120/min.
   c. Oral temperature 98° F. or subnormal 97-98° F.

    d. Tender spot on belly, two inches above and two inches to right of belly button (*see* Fig. 27).

    e. Lower belly gurgles and rumbles.

If more than two of the above symptoms are present, suspect bleeding duodenal ulcer!

1. Put him to bed.
2. Give two ounces of milk or antacid (Gelusil, etc.) every hour until 2300 hours daily.
3. Allow in addition only water or tea with sugar by mouth.
4. Give Demerol 75 mgms (1½ cc or ml) by injection, soon.
5. He may vomit dark "coffee-ground" material. This may precede the black diarrhea. Emesis increases fright. Repeat Demerol 75 mgms (1½–2 cc) every four hours to control apprehension.
6. Patient may have one or several more liquid, black, stinking stools.

The ulcer will usually stop bleeding after 48 hours with the above treatment.

    a. Nausea and emesis subside.

    b. Pulse is slower than 100/min.

    c. Sweating is less or stops.

    d. Apprehension lessens; no Demerol needed.

    e. Black diarrhea stops.

Follow-up treatment:
1. Keep patient in bed.
2. Continue antacids every two hours—1 ounce.
3. Begin bland feedings every four hours: Milk; canned, powdered; soft or boiled eggs; mashed potatoes; rice, oatmeal, tapioca, or macaroni and cheese. As much as the patient wants.

Patient will improve over next 2-3 days. If above diet is tolerated on the 4-5th day after onset of bleeding:

1. Start ulcer diet prescribed for an uncomplicated ulcer.
2. Patient may have dark, but not liquid, stools for several days after other symptons subside.
3. Antacids may produce constipation. Give an enema if necessary.
4. Allow patient to resume activity gradually; he will be weak for several days to two weeks.
5. Bleeding ulcer which fails to stop (i.e., black vomiting and diarrhea continue more than 24 hours) requires sophisticated medical care quickly. Holler for help! Continue treatment until it arrives.

Discussion—Bleeding Duodenal Ulcer

The duodenal ulcer bleeds when it erodes a sizable artery. This does not hurt much because a blood film shields the ulcer base from irritating duodenal contents.

Blood in the gut produces dramatic symptoms. In the stomach hydrochloric acid converts it to acid hematin. This looks like old coffee grounds and is very nauseating. Violent hematemesis-vomiting of blood follows.

In the lower intestine, whence it is propelled by the peristaltic motion of the bowels, the digestive ferments and bacteria turn blood into a black, gummy foul-smelling mess. This, too, is irritating and a tarry-stool diarrhea follows. A nasty by-product is a considerable amount of gas which can be heard gurgling in the lower abdomen.

Both the systemic response and conditions at the ulcer site combine to protract bleeding.

Hemorrhage anywhere in the body incites a general alarm reaction. The adrenal glands secrete nor-epinephrin which accelerates the pulse, increases the heart output and raises blood pressure.

Digestive enzymes, mainly hydrochloric acid at the ulcer site, repeatedly dissolve clots before they firmly plug the bleeding vessel.

Treatment aims to reverse these adverse effects. The generous use of Demerol allays apprehension and slows circulation. Administration of bland foods or alkalies absorbs acid and allows a firm clot to form.

This is best done early for continued severe bleeding depletes clotting mechanisms and induces a state of general circulatory insufficiency that depresses all defense mechanisms. If you cannot stop bleeding from a duodenal ulcer within 24 hours, you will need outside help because transfusions may be necessary.

In summary then, it is evident that a duodenal ulcer may heal without developing any complications if treated early and thoroughly with rest and diet. As a matter of fact, 80-95 per cent of duodenal ulcers when treated do heal promptly.

Although managing the simple duodenal ulcer on shipboard is troublesome, it is much better than allowing it to go untreated.

It is also true that abdominal pain is usually not serious. But watch it carefully always. Then the occasional case of appendicitis, gallbladder disease, or duodenal ulcer will be recognized for early treatment.

GENITOURINARY EMERGENCIES

One Wednesday, at 1300 hours, a two-pole spinnaker jibe is in progress, and one of the foredeck gang unwisely straddles a pole. The foreguy is freed, and a gust hoists the sail skyward.

The wayward pole crunches his crotch and throws him half overboard. Pulled back aboard, he falls to the deck groaning and holding his smashed testicles.

1. Get him below. He will be weak and in a shock-like condition, pulse rapid, sweating and pale.
2. Put cold packs, ice if possible, on the injured parts. They will swell remarkably.
3. Give him Demerol 100-125 mgms by injection, soon.
4. Raise the race escort vessel by radiotelephone. Indicate that you have a casualty that needs evacuation. Escort vessel reports she is 360 miles from your position. At 10 knots, they will rendezvous with you in approximately 36 hours.

By 2000 hours your patient's penis and testicles swell massively. He passes a few drops of bloody urine with considerable effort and pain.

At 2300 hours he complains not only of lower belly pain but of marked desire to urinate plus inability to pass more than a drop or two of bloody urine.

Break out the prepackaged urethral catheterization tray (*see* Fig. 29). Contents vary, but all brands contain:

1. A Robinson catheter (plain tip) size 14-15 fr.
2. Plastic cups and antiseptic solution.
3. Graduated basin to measure urine.
4. Lubricant for catheter.

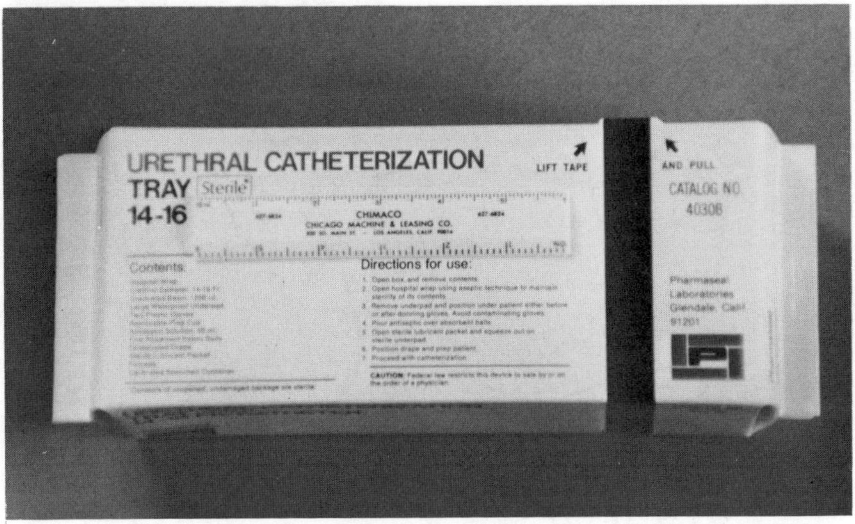

Fig. 29: Prepackaged urethral catheterization tray.

The procedure is:

1. Scrub your hands ten minutes with Phisohex and fresh water sterilized by boiling 20 minutes.
2. Open the prepackaged urethral catheterization tray. Spread out the sterile towel and neatly dump the contents onto this.
3. Put on the sterile gloves.
4. Pour antiseptic solution into one of the plastic cups.
5. Have patient lie flat on his back with knees drawn up.
6. Elevate tip of patient's penis in left gloved fingers.
7. Wipe it well with antiseptic solution.
8. Lubricate tip of catheter. Insert it into the urinary meatus (the outlet in the penis) with right hand.
9. Advance the catheter steadily. Have patient take a series of deep breaths. Keep steady pressure on catheter but do not jab it.
10. The catheter will pop into the bladder. Urine flow indicates catheter is in place.
11. Tape the catheter to the penis, or if you have used a Foley self-retaining catheter, inflate the balloon (*see* Fig. 30).
12. Give Azo-Gantrisin 1.0 gm (2 tablets) at 0800, 1400, 2000, and 0200 hours daily while catheter is inlying.
13. Urge oral fluids. Keep intake over 2500 cc (2½ quarts per day).

You have established urinary drainage and have begun antibiotics to prevent infection. There remains only the usual care of the bunk-fast patient and control of pain.

Swelling and pain of penis and testicles should gradually subside. If the urine is red with blood at first, it will gradually clear.

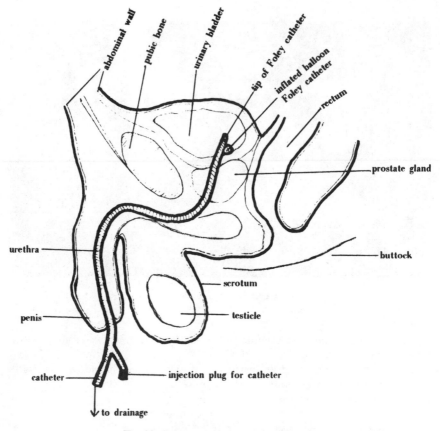

Fig. 30. Foley catheter inlying—side view.

In the unlikely but possible event that:

1. The escort vessel does not arrive in 48-60 hours.
2. The patient is unable to void *any* urine at all.
3. You are unable to pass a catheter.

The bladder will be distended and must be emptied. Complete urinary retention is fatal in 3–5 days.

Proceed as follows:

1. Wash your hands ten minutes with Phisohex and fresh sterile water.
2. Gently percuss or feel the outline of the distended bladder. It will be located in the lower abdomen immediately above the pubis bone (*see* Fig. 31).

3. Wash the abdominal wall over the distended bladder well with Phisohex and sterile water. Paint with antiseptic.
4. Plunge a three-inch spinal No. 18 or other large hypodermic needle straight through the abdominal wall into the bladder. Urine flowing out will tell you when it is in place.
5. Remove as much urine as possible. Suck it out with a big syringe. If you do not have one, simply press on the abdominal wall alongside the needle, being careful not to dislodge it, and the urine will flow out.
6. When you have removed as much urine as possible, withdraw the needle and wipe the puncture wound with an antiseptic.
7. Repeat every 3–4 days until patient voids, catheterization is successful or the patient is evacuated.

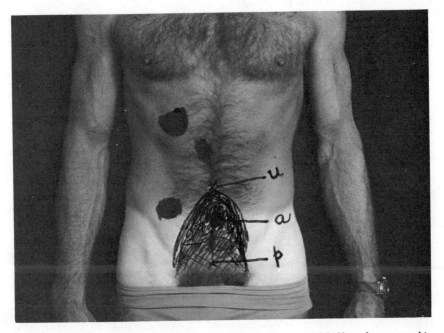

Fig. 31. Location of distended urinary bladder. Do cystotomy at (a) halfway between pubis (p) and umbilicus (u).

Discussion—Genitourinary Emergencies

The serious genitourinary emergency at sea is urinary retention—inability to pass water.

The likely causes are:

1. Local injury to penis, scrotum or perineum (crotch).
2. Reflex inhibition of urination due to non-local injury or severe illness.
3. Swelling of the prostate gland.

Direct injury may transect the urethra—the tube leading from the bladder, through the prostate gland and penis to the outside (*see* Fig. 30).

Swelling of the prostate gland, or other surrounding tissues, may squeeze it shut, even if it is intact.

Rupture of an artery may fill the bladder with big clots that plug the urethra. These will not obstruct passage of a catheter and can be removed by irrigation with sterile water.

Nervous impulses can inhibit voiding and produce reflex urinary retention even though no mechanical obstruction to the urinary tract exists.

Urination by the healthy male demands complex sequential reactions. The start is voluntary; contraction of the urinary bladder which follows closely is involuntary. Control of the sphincter at the bladder outlet is partly voluntary (as when you hold your water through social necessity) and partly involuntary (once the stream is started, it is very difficult to close it off). Finally, the ejaculation of the last few drops of urine is voluntary.

Certain healthy males always go to the end of the line at a public urinal. Nervous inhibition gives them a bashful bladder. Serious illness or injury that requires bed rest and sedation may lead to a similar inability to void.

It is always possible, since there is no mechanical obstruction to the urinary tract, that the patient with reflex retention will void.

The erect position may enable him to urinate; help him to stand beside his bunk.

Eventually the bladder will empty itself automatically. The agony of awaiting this may be more than either of you chooses to endure. But needle cystotomy is not indicated.

Catheterize after 12–18 hours of retention to relieve painful distension. Remove as much urine as possible.

Afterwards withdraw the catheter, urge fluids, and he will probably be able to void spontaneously in a few hours.

If you have to catheterize him a second time, leave the catheter inlying for three to four days.

Give 1.0 gm Azo-Gantrisin (2 tablets) four times daily for three days after a single catheter passage. Give same dose of same drug daily while catheter is inlying and for two days after its removal.

Prostatic infection as a cause of extrinsic urinary tract obstruction with retention is discussed in Chapter VII.

Benign (non-malignant) enlargement of the prostate may produce retention in older men. The onset is gradual over a long period. First symptom is nocturia—getting up at night to void followed after some time by partial retention with frequent spillage of small amounts. Unless retention is complete do not pass a catheter—the individual will maintain satisfactory temporary drainage by frequent spilling (overflow incontinence) of small amounts of urine.

If retention becomes complete then attempt catheterization. You may have difficulty. If you fail, you will have to do a needle cystotomy every 48–50 hours until patient is removed from your care. Use antibiotics as for other catheter procedures.

One final word about bladder infection—acute cystitis. It is much more common in women; causes fever, chills, and frequent, painful urination but never urinary retention.

A course of antibiotics similar to that described for *Prostatis* in Chapter VII will relieve it in four to five days.

Should urinary retention occur, passage of a catheter in the female is much simpler than in the male. Her urethra is much shorter and less subject to obstruction. The only problem you encounter is finding the urethra. It is forward, just behind the clitoris.

SUMMARY

This chapter presents:
1. Minor causes of abdominal pain—management.
2. Major causes of abdominal pain—management.
   a. Appendicitis acute.
   b. Cholecystitis acute.
   c. Duodenal ulcer, simple and with complications of bleeding and/or perforation.
3. Diagnosis and treatment of peritonitis following ruptured appendix, perforated ulcer or other intra-abdominal organ.
4. Common genitourinary emergencies.
   a. Urinary tract injury.
   b. Causes and treatment of urinary retention.

Chapter VII
THE USE OF ANTIBIOTICS

On November 8th the 28-foot sloop *Wa* left Mahe, Seychelles Islands, starting on the second half of a circumnavigation. Aboard were Pete, Addie, and their cat, Coco. Mocambique Island—the next landfall—lay 1,500 miles south and west beyond a belt of calms, contrary winds, erratic currents and generally miserable sailing. Five days later, still 400 miles away from Mocambique, a 40-knot gale blew up, dead on the nose.

At 0900 a huge wave swept the steering vane overboard. It dragged behind as *Wa* lifted and dropped on the 25-foot waves. Pete spent a frantic hour thrashing around on his belly over the tiny fantail to bring the damn thing back aboard.

At 1900 the wind dropped to 20 knots and hauled to the quarter. Pete and Addie started 3-on and 3-off watches to steer by hand in the confused and tumbling seas. Addie relieved Pete at 1200. He went aft to void but was unable to pass more than a few drops of dark urine that burned like fire. Shortly afterwards he had a shaking chill. His temperature was $102°$ F. oral.

Pete drank as much water as he could for the next three hours but still was unable to pass more than a few drops of urine at a time, although he had a growing urge to void. Dull throbbing pain grew more intense at the base of his scrotum and radiated into the small of his back.

He managed to stand his next watch from 1600 to 2000, but felt "a little fuzzy" during the last hour. Addie stood by to prevent a flying jibe.

By 2100, the urge to urinate generated a massive ache through his lower abdomen, lower belly, and down the inside of both thighs. His teeth chattered with pain and fever. Still he could not void.

So Pete held the tiller while Addie went below and broke out the presterilized catheterization set. She took over the helm and Peter catheterized himself (technique described in Chap. VI).

The process, he reported, was "mighty uncomfortable," but the relief, after he had drained away nearly a quart of dark, cloudy urine, was "worth it."

When the catheter was placed in his bladder, he inflated the balloon (*see* Fig. 29) and left it there since he was not sure that he could void and the passage of the catheter one time was all he wanted to undergo.

At 0200 he unclamped the catheter and drained a pint of dark urine. He had another chill. His temperature was $101.2°$ F. The pain of urinary retention was relieved but he still had considerable discomfort at the base of the scrotum and down the inside of both thighs.

He had a urinary tract infection probably related to the irregular eating and drinking, exposure, and local trauma as he lay extended over the cockpit trying to salvage the steering vane. This urinary tract infection swelled the prostate gland, which in turn shut off his water.

To treat this, he took four 0.5 gm tablets of Azo-Gantrisin at 0200, then two 0.5 gm tablets at 0400, 0800 and every four hours thereafter for the next five days. He drank two large glasses of water with each dose of the pills.

By 1000, 13 November, (after 30 gms total Azo-Gantrisin) his pain was relieved. His temperature was 99° F., and he had lost "the fuzzy feeling."

Wisely, however, he continued to take Azo-Gantrisin and drank two glasses of water with each dose throughout the interval recorded above. By the 15th of November he had no distress. On this day he removed the inlying catheter and was able to void readily with only a slight residual burning.

Exposure, irregular voiding, dehydration due to poor eating and drinking conditions, plus the knocking about on a small (or large) boat may produce urinary tract infections. As in this case, the prostate gland may swell and cut off urine flow. Catheterization prevents severe and possibly fatal complications.

Urinary tract infections are common in women, too. However, rarely do they cause urinary retention because the female urinary tract from the bladder to the outside world is very short and there is no structure lying about it which can swell and close it off.

Pete's diagnosis was based upon fever above 101° F., which suggested infection and the symptoms relating to the genitourinary system which localized this infection.

PNEUMONIA

After five months visiting in Nuku Hiva, Pete and Addie left for Penrhyn, about 1,100 miles to the west. The wind vane was repaired and there was no need to keep watches. Nonetheless, at 0530 on 2 May, Addie got drenched by a sudden shower because she was meditating while watching for the tropic sunrise. She finished her watch, but she was shivering and uncomfortable when Pete relieved her at 0800.

She came on watch again at 1200; but felt miserable, "ached all over," and her throat hurt. She stood the watch but about halfway through she began to cough and her chest hurt when she did so. Her temperature was 100° F.

At 1500 she was resting in her bunk and had a shaking chill. The cough became worse and she produced some yellow sputum. She felt short of breath and when she tried to take a deep breath her left ribs hurt. Her temperature at this time was 103° F. Pete noted that her nostrils flared with her rapid breathing, 28 times a minute, whereas normal resting breathing is ten to twelve times a minute.

Addie had acute pneumonia.

Pete got the A.P. Bicillin, a sterilized prepackaged syringe (see Fig. 32), a bottle of sterile water, cotton and antiseptic.

1. He wiped off the stopper on the sterile water and drew 10 cc of water into the syringe.
2. He injected this into the bottle of A.P. Bicillin powder and shook it until it was entirely dissolved.
3. He drew 600,000 units (1 cc) of A.P. Bicillin into the sterile syringe and injected this into Addie's right thigh muscle (see Fig. 7).

Twelve hours later, Addie's temperature was normal and she felt much better. She was well enough to stand watch. Pete advised follow-up treatment with oral penicillin tablets of 250 mgs every six hours for four or five days, to prevent a recurrence of the infection. Addie protested that she "felt fine" and "didn't want to take pills." She would have been wiser to do so.

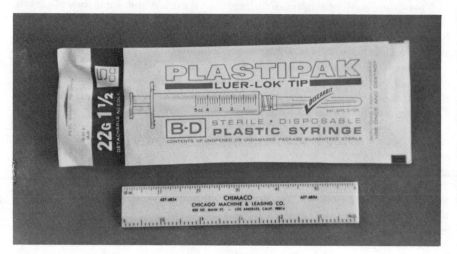

Fig. 32. Sterile prepackaged syringe and needle.

Twelve hours later she had another chill and her temperature following this was 104° F.; symptoms all returned.

Peter gave her a second injection of 600,000 units of A.P. Bicillin. This did not help very much. By May 3rd her temperature was 100° F. at 0800 hours and 103.6° F. at 1600 hours. She felt weak, breathed fast, and her cough hurt more.

May 4th she was about the same or worse. Pete repeated the injection of A.P. Bicillin but this time doubled the dose to 1,200,000 units.

May 5th she felt no better. Peter gave her an alcohol sponge in her bunk which brought her afternoon temperature down to 102° F., but she still felt weak and sick and it hurt to cough.

On May 6th, Pete gave her A.P. Bicillin by injection 1,200,000 units and added Sulfadiazene 2 gms (four 0.5 gm tablets) by mouth and repeated a one-gram dose every four hours. She drank two glasses of water with each dose.

May 8th her temperature was again normal and she felt much stronger although she still had a cough which was productive. Pete continued the same medicines and by the third day she felt well again, although she was somewhat weak,

This time Pete prevailed. He changed to oral penicillin PenVK, 200 mgms, every six hours and continued this with the Sulfadiazene 1 gm (two tablets) every four hours until she had had a normal temperature for two days. (Actually 24 hours was enough, but he was taking no chances.)

Then Pete gave oral penicillin and Sulfadiazene every eight hours instead of every four for one more day. Her temperature remained normal so he stopped all drugs. This time Addie stayed well, although she was weak until they arrived at Tarawa.

Pete is not a physician. However, his management of these two serious infections they encountered illustrates the basic rules for treatment of infectious diseases with antibiotic drugs.

Simply stated, the rules are:

1. Use antibiotics only for serious infections.
2. Select the antibiotic you guess will be most likely to kill the attacking bacterium.
3. When you select the proper drug, be sure the patient is not allergic to it. Ask him; he will probably know. If he is allergic to it, you must use another drug.
4. Give the suggested dose at the proper intervals. Expect dramatic improvement (lowered fever; feeling much better) within 24-36 hours.
5. After the patient's temperature is normal, continue the same dose at same intervals for 24 hours longer.
6. Then reduce antibiotic drug dose to one-half the amount given at the same intervals as before for another 24 hours.
7. If the patient's temperature remains normal on the half dose, stop the medication. If the patient's temperature starts to rise on the half dose, resume the full dose of antibiotic and repeat Steps 4 through 6.
8. If there is no original dramatic improvement in the patient's condition (Rule 4), do one of two things (Pete did both):
   a. Double the dose of antibiotic being given for 24 hours.
   b. Give standard dose of second antibiotic while continuing the first for 24 hours.
9. In either event, unless the patient shows dramatic response to either double dose or double drug within 24—36 hours, stop giving these antibiotics.
10. If you have a third antibiotic, you can now start all over again with Rule 1 and the new drug. Give each antibiotic in standard doses at the proper intervals.

Many diseases that produce high fever are not responsive to antibiotics, so after a reasonable trial as outlined above, stop antibiotics.

Use the chart (see Fig. 33) to select the most likely antibiotic as given in Rule 2. However, if the patient has a high fever and symptoms are indefinite or you cannot decide, try the antibiotics. The chart is only a rough and ready rule of thumb to help you in your selection. Try it on your own if the chart does not answer your specific questions.

Remember, too, that most infections you encounter will never be severe enough to require antibiotic treatment. Common colds are not responsive; most diarrheas are mild of virus origin and require only Bismuth and Paregoric, one teaspoonful after each loose stool, or Lomotil and a light diet for a few days. The other mild infections you will see will subside after a day or two of rest and light diet. Save the antibiotics for the severe infections.

Blood poisoning is discussed in Chapter III on the follow-up care of wounds.

Discussion

Follow these rules to use the antibiotic drugs to best advantage. A physician

ANTIBIOTIC SELECTION CHART FOR COMMON INFECTIONS

Fever 102° F.+ with or without chills		
Local symptoms	Likely disease	Treatment
1. Cough, chest pain, labored breathing, yellow sputum.	Bronchitis or pneumonia	A.P. Bicillin 1,200,000 units by injection. Oral penicillin 250 mgms every 4 hours until infection controlled. Rules 4, 5, 6.
2. Earache—pain when earlobe pulled down.	Otitis media middle ear infection	Same treatment as pneumonia
3. Sore throat—hurts to swallow. Throat fiery red—may have yellow spots on tonsils.	"Strep" sore throat	2,000,000 units (2 cc) A.P. Bicillin by injection daily for 2 days.
4. Frequent and burning urination; urgency.	Cystitis (bladder infection)	Azo-Gantrisin 1 gm (2 tablets) every 4 hours until controlled. 2 glasses of water with each dose.
5. Symptoms of 4 plus pain in back and tenderness between lowest rib and spine.	Pyelonephritis (kidney infection)	Continue Azo-Gantrisin—add ampicillin 250 mgms by mouth every 6 hours until controlled. Rules 4, 5, and 6.
6. Swollen testicles— pain at base of scrotum	Epididymitis Prostatis	Tetracycline 250 mgms by mouth 4 times a day until controlled—0800, 1200, 1600, 2000 hours.
7. Discharge from penis, without fever, exposure	Gonorrhea	Penicillin 2,000,000 units daily for 5 days.

Figure 33.

shoreside with a laboratory available might take a culture of the infecting bug and test it for sensitivity to various antibiotics before he starts treatment.

However, this takes a day or two and often he will begin treatment with the drug of his choice simultaneously. Pediatricians do this often because infections progress rapidly in children; veterinarians usually do it.

At sea you gauge successful treatment by the patient's response. A fever thermometer measures this best. You should take several in metal cases.

Body temperature stays constant in health with a two-degree daily variation that relates to activity. Highest daily temperature is usually at 1600-1800 hours and the lowest at 0300-0400 hours.

This explains why the midwatch is such a bore. Not only are you chilly and alone while the rest of the world sleeps warm and comfortable below, but your body temperature is at its lowest ebb.

How does heat regulation relate to a person with an infection?

Systemic infections constrict the surface blood vessels and drive blood into the deeper tissues where heat loss is diminished.

The infected person first feels his skin cold; he has a chill.

84

Heat production continues and body temperature rises. Shortly a new balance between heat production and heat loss is established at a higher temperature.

Now the patient feels warm all over; he has a fever. It is nature's way of fighting infection. The elevated temperature accelerates antibacterial antibody production.

Severe systemic infections that require antibiotic treatment may develop quickly or slowly.

It was obvious that Addie, who developed shaking chills, a fever of 103° F. in a few hours together with chest pain and cough producing yellow sputum, had a severe bronchitis and/or pneumonia. Penicillin in standard doses was given quickly.

Recurrence of her pneumonia shows the error of stopping treatment too soon. A few hardy germs still lived in her lungs and renewed the attack. It was necessary to add another antibiotic (Sulfadiazene) to the penicillin to overcome this new growth of penicillin-resistant germs.

It is less dramatic when such a fever builds up to this level over two or three days. However, a fever of 103° F. on two successive days, even if it develops gradually, warrants a trial of antibiotic treatment.

You will need more than one antibiotic and more than one form of certain ones to cover the effective range of antibacterial treatment.

Penicillin, tetracyclines, ampicillin and sulfa drugs should be in your First-Aid Kit.

Penicillin for injection (A.P. Bicillin) is stored as powder and dissolved only shortly before use. It deteriorates fairly rapidly once in solution.

Injectable penicillin is useful in raising the blood level quickly in a violent infection. It also may save the day when the patient is vomiting and cannot take pills by mouth.

Ampicillin, which is a penicillin derivative that has a broader spectrum (i.e., is effective against more bacteria), is packaged as capsules for oral administration and also supplied for injection.

Add to the above tetracycline which will attack infecting bacteria not destroyed by the first two.

Penicillin, ampicillin and tetracycline are antibiotics. They are produced by growth of selected moulds similar to those that grow on bread. Penicillin and ampicillin are bacteriocidal; the tetracyclines are bacteriostatic.

There is another type of antibacterial drug, the chematherapeutic. These are chemically synthesized rather than grown and do have antibacterial action.

Sulfanalamide, an analine dye derivative, was the first drug ever to be used in antibacterial warfare. Dogmak, in Germany, introduced this dye in the early thirties.

You will want only two of the multitude of sulfa drugs that overflow the drug stores.

Sulfadiazene (0.5 gm tablets) is given by mouth, readily absorbed and has few unfavorable reactions if given with two glasses of water each dose. It is the drug of second choice in systemic infections. It is often used as adjuvant to penicillin therapy. It is bacteriostatic.

Azo-Gantrisin (0.5 gm tablets) combines a sulfa drug with a urinary tract sedative. It is ideal for treatment of all lower urinary tract infections (bladder, urethra, prostate).

There are hundreds of antibiotic and chemotherapeutic drugs and more are being developed almost daily. If you take penicillin, injectable and oral, ampicillin and tetracycline, as well as Azo-Gantrisin and Sulfadiazene, you will have drugs that cover the useful range of ordinary infections and these will suffice.

Certain other infectious diseases produce almost no fever and yet are best treated with antibiotics.

GONORRHEA

You are four or five days at sea from San Francisco towards Tahiti and your port watch captain shows up one morning with a shameful face, a penile discharge, and complains of great distress when making water.

His last night in San Francisco was "on the town."

1. Examine his penis. Have him squeeze the urethra; pus oozes forth.

The diagonsis is gonorrhea (clap, in the vulgar parlance). This must be treated and since he may have also earned syphilis at the same visit, the treatment must be entended to cover both diseases.

1. Give 2,000,000 units of A.P. Bicillin intramuscularly daily for 5 doses. This will cure both diseases.
2. Should he be allergic to penicillin, then treat only his gonorrhea. Give tetracycline 250 mgms 4 times daily for 5 days by mouth.
3. After either treatment, advise him most strongly to have a blood test for syphilis in three to six months.

Should your port watch captain be a female with the same complaints, the treatment is the same.

DRUG SENSITIVITY

Allergic and sensitivity reactions may appear after any drug administration. You will avoid serious problems by asking the patient if he is sensitive before you give him a drug. Usually he will know. If he is or if there is any doubt, do not give it to him; *you might kill him.*

Immediate drug reaction, called anaphylactic shock, is dramatic and frightening. Shortly after the administration (most often by injection) of a drug, the patient turns pale, collapses and becomes pulseless. He may be conscious or unconscious. Apnea may occur.

1. Mouth-to-mouth resuscitation if needed.
2. Give Adrenalin 1 cc of 1/1000 by injection. Give half of the dose near the site at which the first drug was injected and the other half in another area.
3. Keep patient warm, maintain the level or slightly head-down position.
4. After he begins to recover—color returns, pulse again palpable, sweating stops—give stimulants such as coffee, tea, brandy.
5. If he does not begin to recover within 20 minutes, give an additional ½ cc of 1/1000 Adrenalin by injection.
6. After recovery, keep him in his bunk for 12 hours.

It is well to have ampules of Adrenalin readily available with a syringe for administration whenever potent drugs (antibiotics, etc.) are given.

Delayed drug sensitivity reactions are less awesome although their appearance means all drugs must be stopped except Adrenalin and Pyribenzamine.

Hives are raised—reddish white welts that appear over the body surface and indicate allergy to a drug. They are chiefly annoying because they itch.

1. Stop all drugs.
2. Give Pyribenzamine 50 mgms by mouth every six hours until welts disappear.

Skin rashes also signal drug sensitivity and appear as reddish blotches starting usually on the abdomen and spreading over the whole body. These require the same measures as hives.

Nausea and diarrhea may occur with gastrointestinal allergy to some drugs.

1. Stop the drug.
2. Use Compazine suppositories every 6-8 hours until nausea is controlled.
3. If diarrhea is a problem, give Lomotil tablets two or three times until stools lessen to normal.

If any drug sensitivity reaction, anaphylactic shock, hives, skin rashes or gastrointestinal upsets occur and you have given by injection a long-acting drug, the reaction may continue for some time. After partial recovery, be on the lookout for a recurrence of symptoms and treat it again.

SKIN PROBLEMS

Skin diseases rarely threaten life but they can make it nearly unendurable, particularly in the tropics. At the specific request of the skipper of the *Wa*, whose crew suffered much in this way, a few notes on skin diseases are appended.

The exotic jungle rot fungus and fearsome boils observed in the tropics are essentially the same athlete's foot (dermatophytosis) and staphylococcus skin infections seen in all climates.

The constant moisture and warmth make them grow luxuriantly like all other tropical flora and fauna. Sores become infected easily and heal poorly for this reason; athlete's foot rages wildly beyond the confines of the toes.

Lack of cleanliness also encourages infection, both fungus and bacterial. The first principle then is to keep the skin clean and as free of salt as possible. Wipe the exposed parts at least daily with a small amount of fresh water.

Avoid sunburn, windburn and maceration of skin from prolonged exposure to salt water.

When fungus infection develops, expect it not only between the toes and in the crotch but in the underarms and open sores anywhere on the body.

Daily soaks with Burrow's solution followed by antifungicidal ointment to all areas will heal sores but slower than common in temperate climates. Exposure and drying also help to clear fungus.

Boils and furuncles should have daily antibacterial ointment application and systemic antibiotics (ampicillin 250 mgms 4 times a day for 4-5 days or tetracycline 250 mgms 4 times a day for 4-5 days).

Skin irritations and rashes that produce severe, maddening itching can be controlled by daily application of an ointment containing hydrocortisone.

Resistant ulcers are treated with both antifungal and antibacterial drugs.

Adequate oral intake of Vitamins A, C, and perhaps D, will encourage healing of skin lesions.

Management of wound infections is discussed in Chapter III.

Extensive fungus infections can be helped with daily soaks of ½ or full-strength Burrow's solution.

Vitamin A and D ointment helps to heal resistant sores due to exposure, drying, and salt encrustation.

SUMMARY

Chapter VII presents:

1. Case history of urinary tract infection. Case history of acute pneumonia.
2. Basic rules for use of antibiotic and chemotherapeutic drugs.
3. Chart for selection of proper antibiotic and chemotherapeutic drugs.
4. Mechanism of fever with infectious diseases.
5. Antibiotic and chemotherapeutic drugs.
6. Drug sensitivity.
7. Management of venereal disease.
8. Notes on common skin problems.

Chapter VIII

THE UNCONSCIOUS PATIENT

Force Eight weather catches you somewhere between Newport News and Barbados. Your yawl, *Restless,* running under jib and jigger, bangs into a sizeable wave and tosses the navigator headfirst into a bulkhead. He quivers, then silently rolls to and fro across the deck.

1. Be sure he is breathing. Resuscitate him if he is not.
2. A complete examination (*see* Chap. I) shows the following:
   a. A large lump on the top of his head.
   b. No response to questions; thumb pressure on the eyebrow elicits a groan—he doesn't brush your thumb away.
   c. Both eye pupils are dilated widely and do not contract when a strong light is shone directly into them.
   d. His arms and legs are flaccid—lift them; let go; they flop back to the deck.
   e. The remainder of your examination finds no injury.

The navigator has a severe head injury. You will have to keep him alive until his brain recovers. This is the order of priority:

1. Maintain an open airway.
   a. Keep his head a foot lower than his body. If he vomits, then he won't aspirate the material into his lungs and drown.
   b. Use a bulb syringe, a rag, or your finger to clear mucus, vomit, or his tongue out of the airway. This is a 24-hour-a-day responsibility. Post a continuous watch.
2. Provide adequate parenteral fluids (salt solution) according to Chapters IV and VII. The basic daily requirement is 1000 cc, not 1500 cc as for other conditions.
3. Pass a catheter (preferably a Foley) and leave inlying. This will keep the bunk dry, for he will be incontinent. It also tells you if your parenteral fluids are adequate. There must be 350-500 cc of urine every 24 hours.
4. Give ampicillin 0.5 gm by injection at 1200 hours and 2400 hours daily for fever over 100° F., or if there is persistent bleeding or clear fluid draining from nose or either ear. Give caffeine and Sodium Benzoate 7½ grs. by injection every six hours for three days.
5. Lash him securely in his bunk. Loosen ties; turn him over and relash every four hours.
6. Log daily at 1200 and 2400 hours:
   a. State of consciousness: Comatose, drowsy, agitated, alert.
   b. Reflexes: Pupil response to light; cough; swallowing (elicit by pressure on Adam's apple); response to pressure on eyebrow. (Does he groan and attempt to push your thumb away?)
   c. Rectal temperature—respiration/min.
   d. Spontaneous, purposeful movements of extremities: Yes or No.

He may recover in hours or days. Your log anticipates this.

1. Return of reflexes. Pupils contract to strong light. Gag reflex returns—touch soft palate with tongue blade or spoonhandle. Cough present—blow smoke in his face. Swallows when you press on his Adam's apple.
2. Purposeful movements start. Pushes your thumb away when you apply painful pressure to eyebrow.
3. Regains consciousness—answers questions. Recovery may be incomplete—he may drift back and forth between consciousness and unconsciousness for a time.

Amnesia for accident and a preceding period may persist; space and time orientation poor at first.

It is safe to let him eat and drink when gag and cough reflexes are active.

Or, he may remain comatose until you make port. In this case, you must keep up your supportive treatment.

Prolonged coma brings certain changes:

1. Increased amounts of mucus plug the airway. Insert a Resusitube—push a catheter through it and suck trachea and pharynx dry as often as needed. Use a bulb syringe; reversed air compressor—your own lips.
2. Constipation can cause fecal impaction; bowel obstruction; abdominal distension; vomiting and death by aspiration. Give an enema every third day to prevent this.
3. Flaccid (paralyzed) arms and legs gradually become spastic and rigid. This makes turning the patient difficult, but he must be turned every four hours to prevent bedsores.
4. If coma persists more than four days, pass a nasogastric tube for feeding and medication. If gag reflex is absent, this will be easy.
    a. After tube is in place, bubble test it. Hold the outer end under water, if it bubbles, the inner end is in the lung. Remove the tube and reinsert so it no longer makes bubbles when the outer end is submerged.
    b. Squirt sugar water slowly (2 tbsp. sugar dissolved in a quart of water), two ounces every hour from 0800 hours to 2400 hours daily into the tube.
        Clamp or tie it off between feedings.
    c. If "b" is tolerated, add milk, eggs, mashed potatoes—any food that can be liquefied and passed through the tube.
    d. Note: If patient retches or vomits at any time, get his head low, suck out the airway, empty the stomach through the nasogastric tube.
    e. Check the tube (bubble test) before each and every feeding.
    f. Give antibiotic medication with tube feedings.
    g. Less subcutaneous fluids are needed when tube feedings start. Stop subcutaneous fluid injections when tube feedings produce 500 cc of urine in 24 hours.
    h. Wash mouth out daily with toothpaste, mouthwash, lemon juice or Vitamin C tablets dissolved in water.

Or, patient's condition may deteriorate. Early, this is due to primary brain injury. Later, it may be due to continued bleeding into the brain, infection of the brain, pneumonia, urinary retention or bladder infection.

1. Periods of restlessness, irrational behavior at times alternating with coma or

steadily deepening coma indicate further brain damage. Rising rectal temperature, 103-106° F., also indicates complications.

2. Irregular breathing—periods of rapid, deep breathing alternating with periods of complete apnea (Cheyne-Stokes respiration) indicates severe brain damage.
3. Shallow, rapid respiration with flaring nostrils and cough suggest pneumonia.
4. Cloudy urine may mean bladder infection. Pus extrudes from the urthral meatus about the catheter after it is inlying a day or two. It is no reason to remove catheter. Wipe away discharge with antiseptic solution as needed.
5. Plug-up of the bladder catheter may occur.
6. Dilation of one pupil that fails to contract to light suggests severe damage to that side of the brain. Bilateral persistently dilated pupils that do not contract to strong light indicate severe bilateral brain damage.

You cannot accurately assess the original or continuing brain damage or diagnose certainly which complications are developing. So you must treat all shotgun-like if your log shows the patient is worse.

1. Check airway; be sure it is clear.
2. Irrigate the urine catheter; be sure if flows freely to and fro.
3. Double the dose of antibiotic or add a second drug (see Chap. VII).
4. Give caffeine and Sodium Benzoate 7.5 gms by injection twice daily.
5. Give Decadron 4 mgms (1cc) by intramuscular injection every six hours for three injections.
6. For restlessness or delerium (difficult behavior to control) give Valium 10 mgms by injection, once only, each 12 hours.
7. Maintain necessary restraints to keep patient from hurting himself.
8. For rising temperature (above 105-106° F. rectally), remove all clothing and bedding. Give repeated alcohol or cold-water sponge baths.

Two other conditions may follow a blow on the head, both dangerous but fortunately rare.

A middle meningeal artery syndrome follows a severe blow on the side of the head. There is usually a brief period of unconsciousness followed by apparent recovery. However, over the next few hours, the individual becomes confused, complains of severe headache, loses consciousness, develops deepening coma and usually expires.

The blow has fractured the skull and torn the middle meningeal artery which lies under the bone. Continued arterial bleeding produces increasing pressure which leads to death.

Treatment consists of boring a hole in the skull (trephination) to let the blood out and relieve pressure.

Diagnosis can be suspected if one pupil dilates while the opposite one contracts to strong light.

Subdural hematoma, a syndrome produced by tearing of one of the veins in the meninges (the membranes surrounding the brain), is even more subtle. The original injury is often so slight that it is forgotten. Weeks or even months later, headache develops, followed by irrational behavior and finally, if untreated, coma and death.

Treatment for this condition is trephination.

Discussion—Head Injury

In addition to head injury, diabetic coma, insulin shock, uremic poisoning, drug overdosage, cerebrovascular accident (stroke or brain hemorrhage) or prolonged anoxia (as in near drowning) may produce coma.

Head injury is the most likely cause you will encounter. The unconscious patient is more helpless than a newborn babe whose squall at least attracts attention to discomfort or danger.

Successful treatment of coma demands vigilance and initiative. Do not despair; patients have completely recovered after 29 days of profound unconsciousness.

A blow on the head (or jaw) may stop all brain function briefly. Joe Louis' boxing opponents learned this the hard way. For a minimum of ten seconds they were "out."

Vital functions—breathing, heartbeat, temperature control—returned in seconds; voluntary protective movements, in seconds to minutes; consciousness and coherent thought, in minutes to hours or sometimes days.

Concussion is poorly understood. The brain appears essentially unchanged to the naked eye and under the microscope. Complete interruption of service occurs while circuits appear normal.

If concussion is the only injury to the brain, consciousness returns in a few minutes. A headache may persist for one to three weeks. Rest, aspirin or Emperin and Codeine will control this.

A harder blow may cause, in addition to general concussion, local damage to brain tissue, on the side struck or contra-coup, the opposite side where transmitted force has banged the brain against the skull.

A brain bruise forms like a hidden black eye. It differs from a real black eye in that the skull sharply limits swelling. Instead, the brain presses against bone and raises the pressure within the cranium (intracranial pressure) and squeezes blood out of its own tissue.

Various regions of the brain differ in their sensitivity to oxygen lack. First to quit working is the cerebrum—controlling the thinking and voluntary movement centers.

Increasing cerebral anoxia produces first irrational behavior, then semiconsciousness (patient asleep but can be aroused), finally deep coma, during which no purposeful movements take place even to remove painful stimulation (thumb pressed hard on an eyebrow) and patient cannot be roused.

The vital brain stem (base of brain) centers that control breathing, circulation and body temperature are more resistant to anoxia. They go about their daily tasks, albeit sometimes fitfully, with an oxygen supply that will not keep the sleeping cerebral cells awake.

Failure of these centers indicates severe brain damage.

The respiratory center, in the brain stem, has two chemical controls. Most sensitive is its response to small increases in carbon dioxide in the arterial blood. When you walk a little faster, your muscles make a bit more carbon dioxide (within seconds this circulates to the respiratory control center), you breathe harder and blow off the excess carbon dioxide; slow down and within seconds your breathing is back to walking normal.

The second control—response to lowered oxygen content in arterial blood—is far less sensitive. Violent exercise (running the quarter mile) demands so much oxygen for muscle function that the lungs cannot keep up the supply; it also produces more carbon dioxide than can be readily blown away. An oxygen debt and carbon dioxide excess results which you pay back by panting for several minutes after you stop running.

Anoxia following head injury decreases the sensitivity of the respiratory control center to carbon dioxide. Apnea stops respiratory exchange in the lungs. Carbon dioxide content of the blood rises, but the depressed respiratory center will not respond, oxygen content decreases; finally the combination overcomes the sleepy respiratory center. An oxygen debt and carbon dioxide excess, very like that following violent exercise, now make the unconscious patient pant. Shortly carbon dioxide drops and oxygen rises to normal levels. Apnea again develops. The cycle goes on. This is Cheyne—Stokes respiration—an eponym for those physicians who described it. It is a very grave prognostic sign following head injury.

The center for circulation control, located also in the brain stem, responds more favorably to increased intracranial pressure following brain injury. It slows the heart rate (greater filling occurs between beats), stroke volume rises and increases systemic blood pressure in an effort to force more blood into the crowded, gasping brain cells.

The temperature control center is resistant to anoxia so marked changes in body temperature denote severe brain injury. Heat loss mechanisms (seeChap. V) fail; the temperature rises rapidly. If the center does not recover, body temperature of 107-108° F. may cause irreparable brain damage.

The severity of the original injury will determine the degree of increased intracranial pressure and brain dysfunction. If the hurt is not too great and if you support the vital functions, eventually brain swelling will subside, the neurons will heal, consciousness will return and gradual recovery follows.

The treatment outlined is supportive except for three specific measures. First, Decadron is an adrenal cortical hormone that reduces brain swelling directly; second, the alcohol sponge baths reduce rising body temperature and protect the brain from heat damage until the temperature control center recovers; third, the antibiotics given when there is blood that will not clot, or clear fluid draining from the nose or the ear. Such liquid is cerebrospinal fluid formed in the brain. Its leaking denotes a fracture through the base of the skull. Unless prevented by antibiotics, bacteria may ascend through the cracked bone and infect the brain.

We have said little about fracture of the skull here. You cannot detect its location without an X-ray and, except for the rare depressed fracture, it is of no importance. It is damage to the brain that counts. To my knowledge, there is no tale of a skull that failed to knit if the brain beneath survived.

In summary, if you support brain stem centers that keep respiration, circulation and temperature control working, you will keep the unconscious patient alive until he recovers consciousness.

You treat a patient with a spinal fracture and injury to the cord in much the same fashion. Depending upon the level of injury he will be paralyzed from the neck down (quadriplegic), or from the waist down (paraplegic).

In a cervical fracture, he may be unconscious. This is rare in lower spinal injury. Your treatment will be to supply what you can of those functions that he cannot do for himself. He may have to be fed, have an airway maintained, be given extra fluids, require an inlying catheter just as an unconscious patient does.

He will guide you in what he needs.

DELERIUM AND OTHER BEHAVIOR PROBLEMS

November 6, 1968, *Diastole*, a 36-foot cutter, headed south out of Los Angeles Harbor on the Mazatlan race. Her crew of six included as navigator, Dr. Arthur Stritch, her physician captain, and five others.

Los Angeles was in the midst of an epidemic of Hong Kong flu and poor *Diastole's* crew took the brunt. The weather was fair but she was sailed shorthanded. Dr. Stritch got the flu 24 hours out of port. Two days later, when he had recovered sufficiently to stagger into the cockpit and hold the wheel in a brave simulation of watch standing, two other members were flat on their bunks. And so it went.

Some 700 miles downwind, the midwatch got a squall; the spinnaker filled the *Diastole* began to run. The watch, two of the walking ill, saw the youngest crew member crawling up out of his bunk to the stern pulpit.

Suddenly there was a wild burst of screaming and singing audible even above the whistle of the wind. Dr. Stritch turned a flashlight aft. Balanced on one foot on the pulpit, holding to the backstay with one hand and gyrating back and forth, stark-naked and yelling at the top of his lungs, was the youngest member.

With no hope of reasoning with him, Dr. Art jumped up and grabbed the lad as he went wheeling off to port with the ship's roll. After a struggle, he was safe in the cockpit. Or was he? He kept jumping up, eyes rolling wildly. He was in his own private shrieking world; contact was impossible.

The others awakened. They wrestled him below, wiped him dry and wrapped him in a blanket. He threw it off and started topside the moment they let go of his hands and feet. They managed to take a rectal temperature (one man sailed the boat while four accomplished this medical maneuver). It was 107° F. He had the "flu."

Dr. Stritch:
1. Wrapped him firmly in a blanket.
2. Had two crewmen hold him down.
3. Gave him by intravenous injection slowly 10 mgms of Valium. (Intramuscular would have been just as effective. It would have been a few moments longer taking effect, however.)

Twenty minutes later the patient was snoring away as though fever delerium and irrational behavior on a small sailboat in the middle of a squall had never happened.

The next morning his temperature was somewhat lower. He was given a course of tetracycline, 250 mgms every four hours, until his temperature had been normal for one day. It took two days to accomplish this.

He had no further bouts of delerium—and he did not remember his midnight episode.

Discussion

Irrational, uncontrollable behavior is somewhat analagous to scrambling of electrical circuits anywhere. The elements of proper perception of various stimuli and relevant action are lost. Many times stimuli arising from such short circuits project outward sensory impressions which do not really exist (hallucinations).

Anoxia commonly will disorganize the brain patterns of reception and response. This is most likely due to loss of cerebral (controlling) function while the motor centers are still relatively intact. Such anoxia may result from high fever which demands so much oxygen for the body that the brain is in short supply. Or high temperatures may directly disorganize the brain cells themselves.

Drugs of various types will alter cerebral and brain stem function. And at times, withdrawal of drugs (alcohol) may do the same.

Regardless of the cause, unruly behavior that endangers a man must be controlled. In the case described, had the boy not been restrained there is little doubt he would have been lost overboard.

Many times moderate physical restraints will suffice. If some obvious cause for anoxia (a semiconscious patient with a partially obstructed airway) can be found and corrected, this may render the individual tractable.

If it is necessary or is evident from the outset that drug control is needed, Valium or Thorazine are the drugs of choice—probably by injection, although it is possible that patients suffering a mild degree of troubled behavior can be talked into taking it by mouth.

Since the brain is already injured, these drugs should be used cautiously. Start with small doses (2.5–5 mgms Valium) and watch for half to three-quarters of an hour. Then you will not wind up with a patient who is too depressed to breathe and needs resuscitation.

Do not be afraid. Proceed slowly but do continue until you get the desired effect, i.e., a calm tractable or sleeping patient. There is really in the last analysis no dose of a drug, only the amount which produces the desired effect.

Head injury and delerium tremens from alcohol overindulgence are indications for extreme caution in the use of potent tranquilizers. But use them if you must.

Once you gain control, maintain it. Perhaps the cause will pass quickly as it did for the boy with the flu. Watch your patient carefully—the drug will not wear off all at once. You may note signs that suggest you had better repeat the dose after one or two or many hours. Stay ahead of your patient by careful observation.

Chronic anxiety and depressive states that develop on long cruises are beyond the scope of this book. They may cause unpleasantness aboard and interfere at times with peak performance. Excluding the suicidal and the truly psychotic, these conditions are not dangerous.

Proper attention to bowel habits and mild heat exhaustion, simple as it sounds, will do much to make life pleasant for all. Rotation of tasks to relieve monotony is a great morale builder.

Extreme fatigue may endanger all hands under severe conditions. It might be necessary to pump a leaking vessel for days. There have been instances where the strain of this was so great that everyone, or nearly everyone, was ready to quit.

To render the impossible possible, I feel amphetamines should be used. There is little evidence that they improve athletic performance in the properly conditioned athlete under the minor strain of competition, but they do give a psychic lift and when everyone is hopelessly discouraged in a really hazardous situation, they might prove helpful. Dexamyl 0.5 mgm, a mixture of amphetamine and a barbiturate (an upper/downer combination) will give the necessary lift while not rendering the individual too nervous and frightened to be useful.

Such a dose can be repeated at intervals of from four to 24 hours, depending upon individual responses to the drug. This is great; some persons get a five-day lift out of one tablet while others are helped only for a few hours.

It should be used only when very real danger threatens. Things usually look worse at sea than they really are. Use careful judgment in deciding how great the danger and how hard to push the crew.

If amphetamines have been taken over several days, it is well to decrease them gradually, not stop them abruptly. Cut the dose to one half for a day, then to one quarter and finally stop it.

Serious, even suicidal, depression has followed the sudden cessation of amphetamines.

Extreme fatigue arising from long stretches of unruly weather, or the whirring of winches inches above your head during a long race that prevents sleep, raises the question of the use of sleeping pills. In my opinion it is contraindicated.

When you get tired enough, you will sleep—in a wet bunk with the on-watch trampling over your head. And should you be needed for an all-hands maneuver, you will not be drugged and a danger to yourself and your shipmates. Leave the sleeping pills at home.

SUMMARY

Chapter VIII includes:
1. Case illustrating severe head injury.
   a. Management of severe head injury
   b. Follow-up care, including: improving; status quo; deteriorating.
2. Discussion of physiology of head injury.
   a. Concussion.
   b. Brain damage.
3. Management of patient with paralysis from spinal cord injury.
4. Delerium and other behavior problems.
   a. Case illustration of high fever delerium.
   b. Management of high fever delerium.
5. Discussion of irrational behavior.
6. Chronic anxiety and depressive states.
7. Extreme fatigue under dangerous conditions.

Chapter IX

NOTES ON PREPARATION

You love your boat and never sail to far-off waters without a meticulous overhaul. But what about the men who man her? Spare parts are easier to come by than spare crew where you are going. Your moral obligation to the safety and pleasure of the expedition demands maximum preparation of both. Each member of the crew has a complete medical examination. The results should be discussed privately with you.

A chronic disease need not exclude the sufferer but you accept added responsibility. For example your potential port watch captain is diabetic. He has known and controlled it well for years and plans to provide his own medications and care. If you will learn to manage diabetic coma and insulin shock, take him along. If you cannot, replace him. Another has hypertension (high blood pressure) but it is mild and uncomplicated. Do not worry about him except remember he is not the best candidate for an unnecessary stressful task. Duodenal ulcer disease may plague another. Present status and possible complications discussed with the man and his physician assure you an extra supply of Gelusil prevents possible trouble.

These few from a multitude of possibilities illustrate the principle of prevention by preparedness. But what about yourself, skipper? You are the hub about which the whole wheel revolves—have your doctor poke and prod you until he is sure no unsuspected dry rot will collapse you. Ask him his thoughts about an elective appendectomy. If you or any of your crew have gallstones, these should be removed.

Emotional instability leads to problems in long cruises. Unfortunately this is often difficult to predetermine; most physicians are reluctant to expose their patients' neurotic traits.

You will have to do a bit of discreet probing. A background of difficulty in dealing with proper authority, frequent alcoholic binges, numerous changes of occupation and/or wives might make you wonder if a certain fellow is just the man you want on watch as you dodge among the reefs and atolls of the Gilbert Islands.

Most sailor men drink; many drink a lot. In my opinion, it is a question of when a man drinks—when the work is complete, or when he should be sober and on the job. Many times the choice is difficult. Balance personal charm and sailoring expertise against immature irresponsibility of character.

Drug usage is common among the affluent young—just as alcohol usage is common in the older affluent. It is doubtful if you will ever find a hard-core addict (heroin, Demerol, cocaine) seeking a berth for a long ocean race or cruise. But many sailors are frequent marijuana smokers (pot heads) and some use amphetamine (speed freaks).

Your only concern is the safety and pleasure of your cruise. Avoid the popular argument, i.e., is alcohol or marijuana the "safer" drug. Poor timing in the use of any drugs (including alcohol) may warp judgment when it should be keen. Continued excessive use of any drugs (including alcohol) leads to serious defects in judgment and courage.

The argument is practical, not moral. The use of amphetamines is prevalent in the attempt to improve athletic performance. Exhaustive studies at a leading medical school found no evidence to support this theory.

Do not find yourself in the position of the skipper whose forward lookout was drunkenly asleep on watch while the helmsman, high on amphetamines, thought it simpler to sail over San Clemente Island than to tack around the west end.

A balanced diet (protein, calories, mineral and vitamins) is as essential to top crew performance as proper sail trim is to beating to weather. Vitamin C is particularly important since man neither makes nor stores it. Evidence strongly suggests that greatly increased amounts are needed (up to 500 milligrams per day) for maximum emotional and physical performance under stress long before scurvy is apparent.

Certain other hazards threaten the unwary. The first week the non-manual laborer is at sea, his hands will be so sore from handling lines as to make them practically useless. Plan on this.

Don't go up the mast on a single halyard. Don't go swimming without posting a shark lookout. Don't cook with deep fat ever (fire hazard), and don't have boiling liquids on the galley stove in the seaway. The list of donts is endless, but the foregoing ones have been the most frequent offenders.

One word about sanitation. People get smelly if unwashed and, more importantly, often suffer painful boils and other skin infections. Tap your heat exchanger or other engine cooling system for hot water, and wash with germicidal soap twice a week. Or, heat water on the galley stove to sponge-bathe. Brush your teeth to prevent the cavity-inspired toothache.

DENTAL EMERGENCIES
(Alex Okrand D.D.S.)

Two major dental problems arise at sea: severe apical abscess spreading to the tissue of the jaw and neck, and a fracture of the jaw.

Dropped fillings and crowns are painful but not otherwise dangerous. A dental kit, complete, prepackaged with instructions for use, will manage such situations. And, of course, proper dental prophylaxis prior to setting out on a journey will minimize lost fillings.

Broken teeth fall in the category of painful rather than dangerous and pain medication plus a soft diet will prove sufficient.

An apical abscess that extends may produce massive swelling of the cheek (if it be an upper tooth) or of the floor of the mouth and neck (if a lower tooth).

The latter, particularly, may be a real threat, for soft tissues of the neck can swell to block the airway—a condition known as Ludwig's Angina.

Should a toothache and swollen lower or upper jaw develop:

1. Tap the teeth—the sore one will be the source of abscess.
2. Give ampicillin 0.5 gm by intramuscular injection when swelling first appears (see Fig. 7).
3. Continue ampicillin by mouth 250 mgms at 0800, 1400, 2000, 0800, daily until swelling subsides.
4. Give Emperin and Codeine ½ gr or Demerol 1-2 cc (50-100 mgms) every four hours as needed to control pain.
5. Liquid diet.
6. Bunk rest.

7. Prepare salt solution (*see* Chap. IV). Have patient hold this in his mouth against the sore tooth as hot as possible four times daily.

8. Discontinue medications when symptoms subside.

A broken upper jaw causes pain and disalignment of the teeth. Efforts to firmly close the teeth hurt and it will be difficult for the victim to open his mouth wide.

If there is obvious displacement of a segment of the jaw, a reasonable pressure to line up the teeth will do no harm.

1. Liquid diet until eating is no longer painful.

2. Tetracycline 250 mgms 4 times a day by mouth for five days.

3. Emperin and Codeine ½ gr. or Demerol 1-2 cc (50-100 mgms) by injection every three hours as necessary for pain.

4. Stop medications and resume normal diet when pain subsides (2-3 weeks).

Fracture of the lower jaw is complicated by difficulties of immobilization.

1. Give Demerol 75-100 mgms (1½-2 cc) by injection.

2. Attempt to align teeth properly.

3. If there is bleeding from gums at fracture site (compound fracture), give ampicillin 0.5 gm intramuscularly soon and every 12 hours for five days.

4. Fashion a jaw sling bandage to immobilize the lower jaw by fixation against the upper. Make it easy for him to remove in case he vomits.

5. If patient can squeeze enough liquid diet through his bandaged jaw, have him do so. If this is too painful, pass a nasogastric tube (*see* Chap. VI) and feed him a liquid diet with a bulb syringe.

Formula:	a. Powdered milk	4 cups (in water)
	b. Eggs	4
	c. Sugar	4 tbsp.
	d. Vanilla flavoring	

This provides roughly 1000 calories per feeding. Two or three daily feedings will sustain nutrition. Mashed potato, pureed soup—indeed, any food liquid enough to pass down the tube—may be added.

He may develop diarrhea. Give Lomotil tablets 2, or bismuth and paregoric 1 tsp. with each feeding.

6. Discontinue treatment when symptoms subside.

SUMMARY

This chapter presents:
1. Preparation of crew by medical examination.
2. Notes on use and abuse of certain drugs.
3. Dental emergencies
   a. Abscessed jaw.
   b. Fractured jaw.

Chapter X
FIRST-AID KIT

You cannot design a First-Aid Kit that gets all used up. If the medical supplies you must stock were consumed, it would be a catastrophic cruise, indeed.

The quantities of antibiotic drugs recommended are based upon a crew of eight for a cruise of a year or more, presuming each person may require treatment of one severe infection. Overlap and substitution provide a wide margin of safety if an

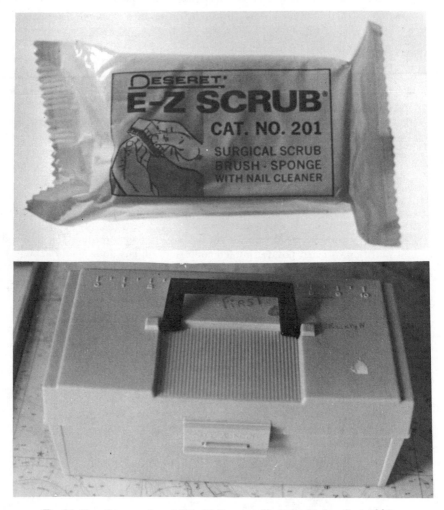

Fig. 34. **Top:** Soap scrub pad. Fig. 35. **Bottom:** Plastic tackle box first-aid kit.

100

unusual number of infections arise. Deterioration of some drugs demands overstocking of the sturdier drugs for the latter part of the voyage, although they are admittedly second choice.

Decadron, Atropine, and Valium, among others you will carry and probably never use. Yet if you do need these they may be lifesaving.

Purchase your drugs and supplies at home before setting out. Consult your physician; he furnishes prescriptions which you must have for many items and, together with your druggist, he may suggest alternate drugs or better methods of packaging than are available at the time of this writing. Finally, familiar drugs travel under strange names in foreign countries. You might not know what to ask for.

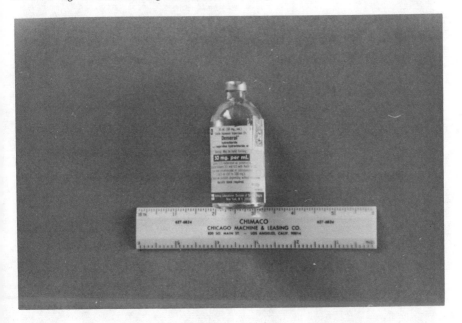

Fig. 36: Demerol—multiple-dose vial 30 cc/50 mgms/cc.

The urethral catheterization kit (*see* Fig. 29), the enema kit (*see* Fig. 26), and dental kit are sterile, sturdily packed and easy to stow. The plastic covers resist moisture so long as the seals are intact. Do not sterilize these for reuse by heat; it melts the plastic. Scrub the instruments well with Phisohex and fresh water, then rinse and soak for two hours in antiseptic such as rubbing alcohol.

Disposable syringes and needles (*see* Fig. 32) and soap scrub pads (*see* Fig. 34) are sterile, prepackaged in water-resistant but not waterproof paper. A glass or metal syringe with metal-hubbed needles should be taken, too, because it can be resterilized forever.

You may have storage for liter bottles of prepared parenteral salt solution; you can make your own if you do not or if a sudden emergency uses your supply (*see* Chap. IV).

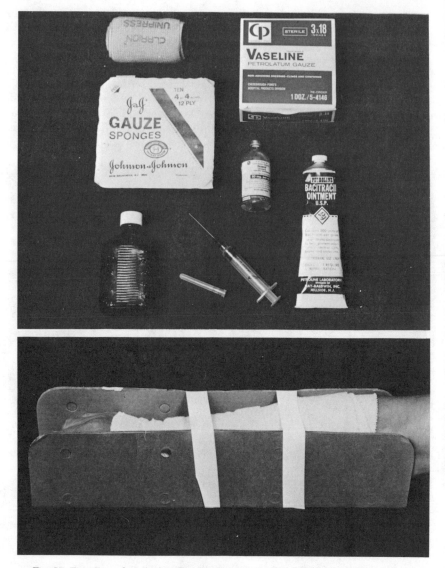

Fig. 37. Top: Burn dressing kit. Fig. 38. Bottom: Cardboard arm splint—stows flat.

We find plastic tackle boxes handy for drug stowage (*see* Fig. 35). There are many sizes—shelves with convenient dividers fold out and the boxes do not corrode.

The following list of drugs and supplies relate only to diagnosis and treatment of the serious emergencies discussed in this book. You will want a standard First-Aid Manual and supply kit for the lesser problems.

All drugs and supplies marked with an asterisk will probably require a physician's prescription.

DRUG LIST

1. Drug and action.
2. Usage.
3. How supplied.
(Bacitracin or Neosporin) 4. Suggested quantity to take with you.

A & D Ointment. Ointment for local application to chronic ulcers.
Supplied as 4 gm tube.

Take: 1 or 2 tubes.

*Adrenalin HCl. Hormone of adrenal medulla. For injection in anaphylactic shock or severe drug reaction.

*Ampicillin. Broad spectrum antibiotic.
Oral use—Capsules 500/mgm capsule.

Take: 50 capsules.

For injection—Ampules 500 mgms (0.5 gm) dry powder + diluent, mix just before use.

Take: 10 ampules
+ diluent.

*Atropine Sulfate. Narcotic—relaxes gastrointestional tract, including the gallbladder.
For injection—1 cc ampules containing atropine sulfate grs 1/150.

Take: 3 ampules.

*Azo-Gantrisin. Sulfa drug plus a urinary tract sedative. For treatment of urinary tract infections.
Oral use—Supplied bottles 100 0.5 gm tablets.

Take: 1 bottle.

*Bacitracin Ointment. Broad spectrum antibacterial ointment for hard-to-heal ulcers or badly contaminated wounds.
Supplied as tube.

Take: 4 gm tube.

Lomotil
*Bismuth + Paregoric. ½ bismuth subnitrate + ½ camphorated tincture of opium.
Supplied in 8-ounce brown bottle.

Take: 1 bottle.

Burrow's Solution. Solution for treatment of severe fungus infections. Topical use only. Supplied in pint bottles and gallon jugs.
For extended tropical cruising, take at least two pints.
Less likely to be needed in cooler climates.

*Caffeine + Sodium Benzoate. Stimulant injection to combat low metabolism following heat exhaustion and after severe head injury.
For injection, sterile ampules 7.5 grs.

Take: 3 ampules.

---

*Prescription necessary.

*Compazine. Potent antiemetic and tranquilizer for use by suppository or injection.
For suppository use—boxes of 6—25 mgms each.

Take: 2 boxes.

For injection—2 cc ampules (5 mgms/cc) boxes of 6.

Take: 1 box.

*Decadron. Potent cortical extract.
Head Injury, shock and venom.
By injection 4 mgms + diluent.

Take: 2.

*Demerol. Narcotic for pain relief (*see* Fig. 36).
By injection—30cc bottles/50 mgms/cc.

Take: 1 bottle.

Ampules—2 cc—100 mgms

Take: 4 ampules.

*Emperin + Codeine. 30 mgms.—narcotic. For pain relief. Less powerful than
Demerol.
Oral—tablets.

Take: 50 tablets.

*Furacin. Topical antibacterial ointment. For burn and wound dressings.
454 gm jar.

Take: 1 jar.

Gelusil. Antacid for treatment of indigestion and duodenal ulcer.
Oral—Packages of individually cellophane wrapped tablets—1000 to a box.

Take: 2 boxes.

Liquid—Bottles of 12 fluid ounces.

Take: 1 bottle.

TAC 0.1%

*Hydrocortisone Ointment. Topical application to severely irritated and itching
skin lesions.
Aristocort.

Take: 1 large tube.

*Lasix. Diuretic. Use after near drowning in SALT water.
10 mgms ampules.

Take: 2.

*Lomotil. Tablets to control diarrhea.
Oral—Supplied cartons 10-100 individually blister sealed tablets.

Take: 1 carton.

*Mycostatin Ointment. For fungus. Topical application.
For tropic cruising.

Take: 2—30 gm tubes.

*Neosporin Ointment. Broad spectrum antibiotic ointment for ulcers, cuts and
onto sutured wounds.
Supplied—1 ounce tubes.

Take: 2 tubes.

Penicillin. Antibiotic for injection and oral administration.
*A.P. Bicillin. For injection—supplied as dry powder (6,000,000 units)/bottle
with sterile water diluent. Mix just before administration.

Take: 1 bottle + diluent.

*PenVK. For oral administration. Penicillin.
Supplied as Redipak (strip pack) 250 mgms—boxes of 100.
Take: 1 box.

*Pitocin. Oxytocic drug. 0.5 milliliters.
Take: 2 or 3,
if females aboard.

(ATARAX)
*Pyribenzamine. An antihistamine tablet used to treat anaphylactic and allergic
reactions to drugs.
Supplied as strip dispenser—50 mgm tablets, 100 to a strip. It is unlikely you
will need a whole strip; 50 tablets should be enough.
Maybe you can split a strip with another skipper.

Sodium Chloride Tablets (salt). Enteric coated.
These dissolve only in intestine and do not cause nausea.
Supplied in bottles of 100. For warm weather or tropical cruising.
Take: 500 tablets.

Non-Enteric Coated. Regular salt tablets to make up salt solution for parenteral
administration after severe burns, shock, peritonitis. Number of tablets needed
per quart will be on the label of the bottle. Take enough tablets to make four
quarts of saline solution. If tablets run out, use 1 scant teaspoonful of table
salt to one quart of water. If you have storage space, take 4 or 5 quarts of
prepared, sterilized salt solution together with tubing, needles + instructions
for use. This may be given subcutaneously, although instructions will probably
suggest intravenous use. Do not add antibiotics to salt solution given
subcutaneously. Antibiotics must be given by separate deep intramuscular
injection. See technique.

*Sulfadiazene. Chemotherapeutic drug for treating infections. Drug of second
choice (*see* chart, Chap. VII). Stores well and does not deteriorate.
Oral use—Supplied 0.5 gm tablets.
Take: 100—0.5 gm tablets.

*Tetracycline. Antibiotic agent for treatment of infections.
Oral use—150 mgm capsules—supplied bottles of 100 tablets.
Take: 1 bottle.

*Valium. Potent tranquilizer for use in controlling irrational behavior from
whatever cause.
For injection—disposable syringes— each contains 5 mgms.
Take: 3 syringes.

Oral use—5 mgm tablets (yellow).
Take: 10 tablets.

*Xylocaine. 1% solution for injection to produce local anesthesia.
Supplied as 50 cc multiple-dose vial—also in 5 cc ampules.
Take: 1 bottle, 50 cc
(10 ampules of 5 cc = 50 cc).

This is a large amount of local anesthetic. However, usage of this amount is
described. Probably 4 or 5 ampules (5 cc) would suffice, except in most
unusual circumstances.

SUPPLIES

Ace Bandage. Elastic bandage for pressure dressing on wounds, sprains, splints. Comes in 2", 3", 4".

Take: 1 of each.

Adhesive Tape. Zinc oxide.

Take: one 3" x 10' roll.

Bulb Syringe. Glass syringe 2-3 ounce capacity with rubber suction bulblike douche syringe or turkey baster.

Take: 1.

Cotton Absorbent. Sterile cotton.

Take: 1 pack.

Bandages. Gauze 1"; 2"; 3".

Take: 6 of each.

Butterfly Closures. Tape strips for wound closure.

Take: 1 can.

Cast Liner. Padding for splints. Also useful for head and jaw bandages. Supplied in rolls.

Take: 2 of the 3" rolls.

Catheter. Rubber tube with fluted tip—to pass through urethra and empty urinary bladder. Retaining balloon—Foley Catheter. Prepackaged sterile.

Take one Foley size No. 14. There will be another (Robinson) in catheter kit.

Dental Kit. Prepackaged—sterile.

Take: 1.

Forceps. Tweezers for various uses.

Take: 1 toothed and 1 plain.

Gauze. 4" x 4" squares—sterile, prepackaged in boxes of 10 (12-ply).

Take: 1/2 dozen boxes.

Graduated Cylinder. Plastic cylinder, measured in ounces and cubic centimeters.

Take: 1 (can also use galley measuring cup).

Hemostat. Artery occluding forceps.

Take: 3 medium.

Kelly Bottle. One-quart bottle with tubing for administration of subcutaneous fluids.
May substitute plastic blood or plasma bottle with proper connections for tubing & needle.

Take: 1.

Knife. Bard (P-a)rker handle No. 3—take one. Blades—sterile packaged in plastic.

Take: 2—No. 10 and 2—No. 15 blades.

Hypodermic Syringes. Plastic disposable prepackaged, sterile—various sizes.
> Take: 4—5 cc with No. 22
> 1½" needle.
> 4—10 cc with No. 18
> 3" needle.

Hypodermic Syringe. Glass, sterilizable 10 cc with metal hub needles. 2—No. 21
1½", 2—No. 18-3".
> Take: 1 syringe and
> 2 each of above needles.

> Note: Some surgical supply houses carry 5—10 cc all-metal syringes. These are
> less fragile than glass.

Cystotomy Needle. No. 18-4" spinal puncture needle.
> Packaged in plastic container.
> > Take: 1.

Needle Holder. Metal forceps with lock handle for holding a curved needle.
> > Take: 1.

Splints. Devices for immobilizing broken bones or crushed extremities. Cardboard;
stow flat and fold up for use.
> > Take: 2 adult.

Pneumatic. Stow flat and are inflated by mouth pressure.
> Take: 1 long enough for upper
> or lower extremity.

Resusitube. Plastic airway for mouth-to-mouth resuscitation.
> Supplied in plastic bag with indelible instructions.
> Carry an extra one in your car. *See* Chapter I.
> > Take: 1.

Rib Belt. Restraint for chest with rib fracture.
> > Take: 1 adult.

Sutures. (Sewing thread) surgical silk or nylon. Packed in individual sterile
envelopes. Swedged onto cutting needle.
> Take: 4 each of 2-0, 3-0 and 4-0.

Steri-strips. Adhesive strips for wound closure instead of sutures. Supplied in
various sizes—6 strips to sterile, plastic package.
> Take: 6 of the ½" x 4"
> and 6 of the ¼" x 3".

Soap Pads. Scrub pads, sterile packaged, individual. Impregnated with antiseptic
soap.
> > Take: 6.

Stomach Tube. Plastic or rubber tube to pass through the nose into the stomach.
Need not be sterile. Should be marked on outer end to indicate location of tip in .
stomach.
> > Take: 1.

Vaseline Gauze. Fine mesh gauze impregnated with Vaseline. Good dressing for burns, compound fractures. Does not stick to wound. Also can make sucking chest wound airtight. Supplied in various sizes, sterile, individual packs.

Take: 1 box of 1 doz. 3 x 36"

Universal Arm Splint. Plastic splint for either forearm and wrist.

Take: 1 adult size.

Thermometer (clinical). To record oral or rectal temperature. Sterilize by wiping off with alcohol.

Take: 3-4 in metal cases.

Thermometer. Wet- and dry-bulb to record relative humidity. Essential for warm weather or tropical cruising.

Take: 1.

The drugs and supplies described on the foregoing pages in this chapter equip a vessel with a crew of eight for a voyage of up to a year. For every boater lucky enough to enjoy such a cruise, there are hundreds—lately thousands—who must limit themselves to weekends or vacation cruises of a few weeks. Such cruises are usually planned within reasonable distance of supervised medical aid.

Here is an abridged list of drugs and supplies which will satisfy major needs of the average cruising or racing sailor. This list, and the supplies on it, are based upon the crew of three or four, and a period of from a few hours to three or four days before medical aid is available.

If you are planning an expedition between the long and short, you can interpolate between the supplies ordered on the previous pages and those presented here.

It is advisable to go over the drug list with your own physician—since many of the drugs will require his prescription. He can show you proper technique for drug injection and with a knowledge of your particular expedition further help to determine the drugs and supplies you'll most likely need.

Following is the list of drugs and supplies presented without explanation of the use or properties of the drugs. They can be found in the original listing on foregoing pages.

DRUG LIST FOR CRUISERS OR RACERS

*Adrenalin—ampule 1 to 1000 (take 2 ampules).

*Ampicillin—(oral capsules) 200 milligrams—take 16 (a 4-day supply).

*Ampicillin—1 multivial plus 10 cc of diluent for injection.

*Bacitracin Ointment—1 large tube.

*Benadryl—50 milligram ampules (take 2). This drug is essentially the same as Pyrabenzamine.

(Drug list for cruisers or racers continued.)

*Benzoin Compound Tincture—take 2 ounces.

*Compazine Suppositories—25 milligrams—take 6.

*Compazine—10 milligram vials for injection—take 3.

*Decadron—4 milligram ampules—take 2 plus proper diluent.

*Demerol—2 cc ampules—100 milligrams each—take 4.

*Emperin and Codeine—30 milligrams—take 12 tablets.

Enema—prepackaged, take 1.

Enteric Coated Salt Tablets—bottle of 100 (only for temperate or tropical cruising).

*Lasix—1 cc ampule (10 milliliters)—take 2.

*Lomotil—take 60 tablets.

*Pitocin—ampules 0.5 milligrams—take 2 or 3 (only if there are females in the crew).

*Tetracycline—500 milligram oral capsules—take 12.

*Valium—10 milligrams in 1 cc ampules—take 2 or 3.

*VK Penicillin—for oral use—take 1 box of strip tablets.

*Xylocaine—1% 5 cc ampules—take 2.

SUPPLIES

Ace Bandages—2- , 3- , and 4-inch, take 1 of each.

Alcohol, rubbing—1 pint.

Cardboard splints—1 or 2 to fit your crew.

Dental kit—1.

Fever thermometers—1 or 2 in plastic or metal cases.

Gauze squares—2 x 4—sterile, 12 to a box—take 2 boxes.

Gauze bandage—1- , 2- , and 3-inch—take 1 or 2 of each.

1 Needle holder

1 Tooth forceps

3 Hemostatic forceps

Plastipak syringes—5 cc, No. 21 needles—take 2.

Prepackaged sutures—3-0 5-0 silk or nylon swedged onto cutting needles—take 2 of each.

Prepackaged Prep Tray—take 1.

Prepackaged sterile vaseline gauze—3 x 36—take 2.

Prepackaged surgical scrub brushes—with antiseptic solution—take 3.

Steristrips—¼ and ½—1 package of each.

Zinc Oxide Ointment—1 tube.

Chapter XI

ABORTION AT SEA

4 June, 0700

Mike and Susie leave Rabaul, New Guinea in their cutter, *Aubain,* round Gazelle Point and head for Thursday Island in the Torres Straits. Distance—1,257 miles—E.T.A. 20 June.

6 June

Susie's expected menstrual period fails to arrive. She's usually prompt. This worries her a bit.

13 June

Susie suddenly has to visit the head every 10 minutes. Her breasts are swollen and slightly tender. She's pretty sure she is pregnant. Mike is both pleased and worried when she tells him.

23 June

They arrive at Thursday Island—pregnancy tests at the hospital confirm the diagnosis. There follow several days of decision making. Doctors are noncommittal as to whether or not they should continue their journey. Finally, Mike decides he can handle *Aubain* alone and they decide to continue their circumnavigation.

1 July, 0700

They head *Aubain* into the Torres Straits to start for Cocos Island in the windy Indian Ocean. Distance—2,761 nautical miles—E.T.A. 27 July.

9 July, 0800

Susie's brushing her teeth—suddenly she vomits. She feels a bit better and stands her watch. There's a good reaching breeze and the steering vane is doing all the work.

1600

She feels better—has skipped lunch, but takes a bit of nourishment now. Mike takes a fix—they have gone 1,044 miles, which leaves 1,717 yet to go to Cocos.

10 July, 0730

Susie wakens violently ill. After vomiting she still feels miserable. Mike gives her:
1. Compazine suppository—25 milligrams.
2. Nausea is only partly relieved, so he repeats this at 1130, 1530, and 1930.

111

11 July, 0003

Susie takes the midwatch.

0230

Susie can't stay awake in spite of coffee and taking off and putting on her clothes. A flying jibe rattles the rigging and tumbles Mike out of his bunk. They heave-to until daylight to check the rigging for damage.

11 July, 0600

Susie's still nauseated—Mike gives her another suppository. She drowses in the cockpit on "watch" while Mike hoists up and tightens the bolts on the starboard spreader tang. He comes down battered but intact and goes below to rest.

1100

Mike takes over the watch. Susie, still drowsy but less nauseated, serves some coffee and biscuits and then folds up on her bunk. Mike stays in the cockpit dozing and waking until 2000, when the wind pipes up a bit. Susie is dead asleep. They heave-to to avoid another flying jibe.

12 July, 0800

Mike takes a fix—250 miles in the past three days, leaving 1,467 still to go. Their poor progress is partly due to fluky winds but also to time lost heaving-to when both are too sleepy to sail.

13 July, 1600

Susie is less nauseated; she takes the watch while Mike organizes a meal.

1700

The wind dies. They flop around in a ground swell. Susie vomits and takes another compazine suppository.

1800

Mike takes the watch till 2400 when he can no longer stay awake, and they heave-to. He remembers saying at Thursday Island that he could handle *Aubain* alone, but he hadn't counted on worrying about a sick wife at the same time.

14 July, 0900

Wind 18 knots, broad reaching, wind vane functions well. Susie feels better and takes some soup.

15 July, 1200

Mike gets a fix . . .348 nautical miles covered since the last position. 1,119 still to go to Cocos.

17 July, 1400

Susie goes off watch, and on her way down the ladder, notes a bit of blood on her bikini—wonders if she isn't going to menstruate after all; a bit late—then she recalls the nausea and pregnancy tests.

17 July, 1800

Susie develops more bleeding from the vagina and dull pain across her lower belly. Mike gives her a Compazine suppository and takes over the watch.

18 July, 0800

Susie has a sudden gush of bloody fluid from her vagina.

2000

Susie's asleep. Mike gets very sleepy and decides to heave-to.

19 July, 0630

Susie awakes with severe cramps across her lower belly that radiate into her back. These come at regular intervals of 5 to 10 minutes and last for a minute or so. She's having steady vaginal bleeding, bright red blood. Mike is concerned, heaves-to and gives Susie:
1. Demerol, 100 milligrams by intramuscular injection.
2. Pitocin, 0.5 milliliters ½ hour later.

1630

Susie's cramps increase, as does her bleeding. After one severe cramp, she passes a large blood clot with a small fetus and membranes.
Bleeding continues though somewhat abated. Mike examines the bloody mess before he chucks it overboard (*see* Fig. 39).
3. Repeats Pitocin, 0.5 milliliters intramuscularly.
4. Demerol, 75 milligrams (1½ milliliters intramuscularly).

2000

"After-pain" and bleeding subside and Susie falls asleep.

19 July, 0800

Susie awakens hungry, thirsty, and with only a tiny show of vaginal bleeding. Mike feeds her and then gets a fix. Somehow in spite of all the difficulties, they have made 150 nautical miles. That leaves a mere thousand, give or take a few miles.

1 August, 1000

Arrive at Cocos Island, clear immigration, and visit the doctor. Good Irishman that he is, he expresses regret at the lost life, but after pelvic examination, pronounces Susie in the best of health.

Later, over a beer, they make a solemn resolve. Birth control pills hold a higher priority in their traveling economy than beer or, perhaps, food.

10 August, 0800

They point *Aubain* westward towards the Seychelles, 2,562 nautical miles across the Indian Ocean. E.T.A., 30 August.

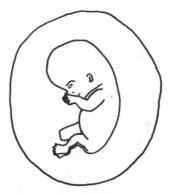

Fig. 39. Eight-weeks' fetus. Actual material passed
may be considerably distorted.

Discussion

Pregnancy is a normal bodily state and usually will go along without serious event. But not always, as Mike and Susie learned.

Frequency of urination is merely an annoying nuisance on a small boat with a crew of two.

Nausea is a common symptom of early pregnancy which usually occurs upon arising, hence the common term "morning sickness." But it may happen at any time. Usually mild, it can be severe enough to require intravenous fluids to maintain water and electrolyte balance.

The cause of nausea and vomiting is a matter of speculation but it commonly occurs during the first weeks of pregnancy.

Surely, the motion of a small seagoing boat aggravates the condition as Susie found out when they flopped around in the large ground swell.

Treatment with Compazine suppositories usually stops the nausea, but drowsiness is a side effect that renders a female sailor ineffective as crew.

Then too, early in pregnancy, drowsiness without any medication often requires many long hours of deep sleep. And, when added to the Compazine effect, makes a really sleepy sailorwoman.

Minimal vaginal bleeding early in pregnancy usually stops spontaneously. Should it persist and increase, particularly if accompanied by tenderness over the lower abdomen and cramps, spontaneous abortion (miscarriage is the lay term) is threatened. A gush of bloody fluid and an increase of cramps, particularly if they are periodic, means abortion is inevitable.

The seagoing treatment for spontaneous abortion is to encourage the uterus to empty itself completely, for this stops further bleeding. An incomplete abortion (i.e., one with retained fragments of the product of conception) may continue to bleed for some time and raises the danger of infection.

This is why Mike gave Susie Pitocin—an oxytocic drug—that induces powerful uterine contractions to expel the dead fetus and membranes. He knew that the uterine contractions produced by the Pitocin would be painful, so he gave her Demerol first.

In this case, it was successful in emptying the uterus and the bleeding stopped and, with the termination of pregnancy, all the other symptoms were relieved.

The bleeding in spontaneous abortion may be considerable and frightening, but it is rarely fatal. Should it continue for long periods, the best that can be done at sea is to replace fluid by mouth and/or by subcutaneous methods (see Chapter IV).

There are many popular ideas as to the cause of spontaneous abortion. Best informed opinion holds it due to defective embryo. And for this reason, Mike and Susie should not feel bad   as the Irish doctor did about the loss of a life. There is no scientific evidence to indicate their situation (i.e., on a sea voyage) had anything to do with spontaneous abortion. It is a medical opinion that a good egg is hard to shake loose.

Many thwarted men and women who have tried illegal abortions by blows to the abdomen and various drugs will attest to that fact.

Douching or other means of emptying the vagina are condemned. The uterus, if encouraged, will empty itself into the vagina and this, in turn, will empty if the woman merely stands up and gyrates a bit.

The pregnant uterus is dangerously susceptible to infection which can be fatal, so stay out of the vagina. Sexual relations should also be avoided for 4 to 6 weeks after spontaneous abortion, and for the same reason.

What are the chances of spontaneous abortion? Statistics show that 10% of all pregnancies end in loss of the fetus—usually from the 8th to the 10th week after conception. In actuality, these statistics are probably low because many early abortions are never seen by a physician. The woman merely believes that she's had a delayed and somewhat heavy menstrual period.

Before the 10th week of pregnancy, the fetus and its membranes are usually expelled intact. Mike was interested—even though somewhat upset by the need to look at it—because he wished to know if it had been completely expelled. It was complete, and he then knew that bleeding would stop. This is the usual course of events.

Finally, this discussion presents no argument for or against contraception by any particular means. It does advise most strongly that no person on land or sea attempt to induce abortion by the use of drugs or any other method, since this can threaten life. In spite of the fact that babies have been conceived and delivered on boats, in hedgerows, in the Outback and at almost any time and place one can imagine, it is better if you are a deepwater voyager to plan to have your child when, for at least 9 to 10 months, you interrupt your journey at a place that furnishes good obstetrical care.

Chapter XII

VENOMOUS VERMIN OF THE SEA; NEAR-DROWNING

0900, September 11th

Pete is snorkeling along the reef at Cocos Island in mid-Indian Ocean. Addie swims nearby. The dinghy they rowed from their sloop, *Wa* (anchored a mile away), is beached. Pete surfaces, feels a sharp stinging across his forehead, then both arms and shoulders. He swims for the beach, some 50 yards away, alerted now and dodging a second Portuguese man-of-war.

0910

Pain clamps his chest muscles tight. He can't fill his lungs. He staggers from the surf, legs wobbling in an exaggerated goose-step and with a wild cry—"Help!"—to Addie, collapses across the dory. He can't move his legs or get a breath.

Addie comes running. Simultaneously she 1) pours a fifth of bourbon whiskey over the welts on his back and shoulders, and 2) begins mouth-to-mouth resuscitation.

0920

Pete's breathing now, though he still can't move his legs. Addie rows the dory and its load back to the *Wa* . She stops twice on the way to resuscitate Pete.

1015

Mike Thurston—whose cutter, *Destiny*, is anchored nearby—sees trouble and comes to help.

Together, they hoist Pete's dead weight (he's still paralyzed) into the cockpit. Mike gets out the medical kit and gives Pete, by injection, 3) Demerol - 100 milligrams; 4) Benadryl - 50 milligrams; 5) Decadron - 8 milligrams. He uses the same syringe and needle for all three injections—does not mix the drugs. And, of course, he washes both the ampule and Pete's skin with alcohol before each injection. 6) Addie slaps a thick paste made of baking soda and seawater on all of the stings.

1045

The paste dries and Addie scrapes the remaining tentacles off with a dull tableware knife.

1055

Pete's breathing well, but deep muscle pain is only partly relieved by the drugs. The stings on his back now begin to burn and hurt.

Addie and Mike heat water in the galley—as hot as they can put their hands in—and dip towels and slap them steaming hot onto Pete. He objects, but they persist. Pain stops and Pete drifts off to sleep in a welter of soda paste, salt water and whiskey.

0800 September 12th

Pete has only slight muscle stiffness in his chest and legs, and a back that looks as though he'd had a taste of the cat-'o-nine-tails (*see* Fig. 40). He's busily putting together an auxiliary first-aid kit to take skin diving. It contains: 1) a resuscitube; 2) a pint of rubbing alcohol; 3) a dull knife; 4) a small package of baking soda; 5) Decadron—8 mgms—two 4-mgm ampules; 6) Demerol—100 milligrams—1 ampule; 7) Benadryl—50 milligrams—1 ampule; 8) 10-cc plastic syringe and sterile needle.

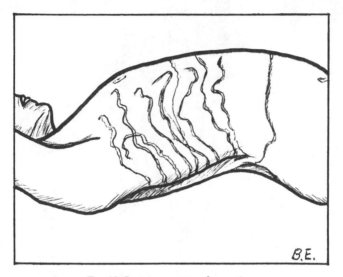

Fig. 40. Portuguese man-of-war stings.

Discussion

The poison of the Portuguese man-of-war and of sea wasps is 75% as toxic as cobra venom. It is less often fatal because the delivery apparatus is less effective than cobra fangs. Nevertheless, extensive exposure is dangerous and can be fatal. The Portuguese man-of-war is not a single vessel, but a whole seagoing colony of thousands of tiny cells clinging to a central floating stalk (*see* Fig. 41). Some members digest the food, some specialize in reproduction, but the dangerous ones are those with the long tentacles, the base of which house the projectile nematocysts containing the poison. The venom can be discharged through the intact skin when the tentacle first attaches itself to the victim or later on, particularly if the nematocyst is stimulated.

This explains why Addie poured bourbon whiskey onto Pete's stings but made no immediate effort to remove clinging tentacles. Alcohol neutralizes the poison already discharged. The baking soda-seawater paste and dull-knife scraping remove those as yet undischarged nematocysts. Rough removal, as with wet sand or a sharp knife, or rinsing these tentacles with fresh water, would stimulate the remaining nematocysts to discharge their toxins. In the event that baking soda is not available, alternating dry sand and seawater can possibly be a substitute.

The toxin is a complex combination of chemicals; 5-hydroxytryptamine (5 Ht for short) is a potent, deep muscle pain-producing substance. The exact mechanism of action is unknown. The best opinion at the moment is that pain is due to sensitization of the nerve receptors by the drug. This drug also causes much of the local itching and burning at the site of the lesion.

Tetraethylammonium hydroxide (tetramine for short), another component of the poison, has a curare-like action that causes the muscle spasm and paralysis. There are, in addition, a number of low molecular weight protein poisons in the compound.

This combination of poisons produces the muscle spasm, paralysis, the bronchial spasm that stops breathing, the shock and collapse, as well as the local skin welts.

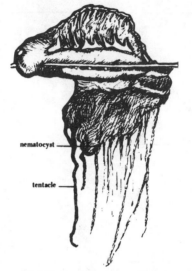

Fig. 41. Portuguese man-of-war.

Demerol is given to control the pain, which in an extensive invenomation is agonizing. Benadryl, an antihistamine, combats the bronchial spasm to aid in breathing and also reduces the severity of the skin welts.

The cortisone Decadron is thought by many to aid in minimizing vascular collapse and shock.

Finally, the compound venom is heat-labile; temperature of 120° F. will render it harmless. The hot towels at 120° F. (which is about as hot as one can stand) do this. You will not burn the skin except on a child before puberty or on the aged.

The cortisone ointment rubbed into the skin welts reduces the inflammation and hastens the healing of these lesions.

It is beyond the scope of this book to consider all of the dangerous creatures of the sea. Sharks, barracuda, and other fishes can produce serious or fatal wounds to swimmers. It is best to maintain a shark watch when swimming in strange waters, particularly between Latitude 25° N. and Latitude 25° S., although attacks by fish do occur in other areas.

Stingrays cause a painful wound that is slow to heal, and (rarely) systemic collapse. The injuries occur most commonly when a swimmer dashes into the surf and steps on a stingray buried in the shallows. "Go easy in on strange beaches" is a good motto.

Spiny urchins do not attack unless touched or stepped on. Be careful of strange-looking rocks when swimming or diving.

A final word of caution. There are, particularly in the coral reef areas of the world, many fishes that are poisonous to eat. Captain Cook described them many years ago and James Bond brought them to literary fame when he was nearly fatally poisoned by the venom of a puffer fish.

If you plan an extended cruise, particularly in southern waters, and expect to eat what you catch—best you learn what is good and what is bad, ichthyologically speaking.

NEAR-DROWNING

Drowning contributes the most deaths from water sports. If you fish a near-drowned person, unconscious and not breathing, from the water, you must instantly institute mouth-to-mouth resuscitation. Seconds count! Don't waste time trying to empty the stomach, the lungs, or move the individual to a better location.

1. Elevate the jaw.
2. Clear the airway of tongue, mucus, mud, and so forth.
3. Close the nostrils with one hand.
4. Place your mouth over the victim's mouth, take a deep breath and blow it into the lungs.
5. Remove your mouth—exhalation is automatic.
6. Repeat 10 to 12 times per minute (15 to 18 times per minute if a child; also, put your mouth over both nose and mouth of a child).

When consciousness with normal breathing returns, watch the patient carefully for at least 8 hours.

If difficult breathing and/or collapse recurs, re-resuscitate at once. Also, give by deep intramuscular injection:

1. Decadron—8 milligrams (two 5 cc ampules). If patient is a child under 10, give 4 milligrams, or one ampule.
2. If near-drowning occurred in **salt** water, give by injection Lasix (furosamide)—10 milligrams (one ampule). (If individual is a child below 10 years of age, give 5 milligrams (½ ampule)). If near-drowning occurred in fresh water, omit the Lasix (furosamide).

The delayed collapse, which may occur up to five to six hours post-accident, is due to water aspirated into the lungs at the time of near-drowning. Ocean water is hypertonic due to its salinity. It draws fluid from the bloodstream into the alveoli by osmosis. This is pulmonary edema and interferes seriously, even fatally, with oxygen and carbon dioxide gas exchange in the lung. It may cause frothy sputum with noisy breathing.

The massive dose of corticosteroid (Decadron) aids the body defense mechanisms to overcome this hazard. The furosamide (Lasix) is a diuretic—it prods the kidneys to excrete water. This reduces the blood volume rapidly and helps dry out the lungs.

Fresh water, on the other hand, is hypotonic; the osmotic force works the other way to absorb water from the lungs into the bloodstream where it dilutes the chemicals in the blood and leads to serious electrolytic imbalances usually manifested by circulatory collapse. It is unwise to give the diuretic Lasix here, because this causes increased loss of electrolytes which are already dilute. The corticosteroids (Decadron), however, do help the body mechanisms that strive to correct the circulatory and chemical imbalance.

The antibiotic, Ampicillin, acts to prevent a postaspiration pneumonia in either type of near-drowning.

After primary resuscitation, when consciousness returns and the patient's breathing has resumed, it is best to get the near-drowned person to a hospital. Oxygen, mechanical ventilators, laboratory tests for blood oxygen, carbon dioxide, as well as blood electrolytes, may be needed to manage a given case.

However, if such help is unavailable, the advanced first-aid treatment here outlined can tip the balance in the patient's favor. It will do no harm.

Chapter XIII

MEDICAL PROGNOSIS—A USEFUL ART FOR SAILORS

You are cruising Baja near Magdalena Bay in your trawler, *No Sudor*, with your wife, 18-year-old son and 16-year-old daughter. A sudden lurch pours a kettle of boiling soup onto your wife's chest and abdomen, or perhaps tosses your daughter through an open hatch to break an ankle. Or possibly, on a sparkling Tuesday morning, son John skips morning chow—an unusual event—and complains of a bellyache.

Unpleasant to think about, yes. Like storms at sea, accidents and illnesses, though rare, do occur. And just as good seamanship will get you through a major blow in the best possible shape, so some knowledge of what to expect from a particular illness or injury will bring you and your crewman through in the best possible condition.

Medical prognosis is the art of predicting the future course of a given accident or illness. It's useful for the cruising or racing skipper. Although difficult, if background information is applied with the courageous common sense usually displayed by deepwater sailors, it will help when trouble comes.

This chapter provides such information in everyday terms. It won't make you a doctor, but it may help you in the same way that an engineering manual will help you start your stalled *Atomic-4* far out at sea.

This discussion provides no treatment for any particular sickness or injury. Details of emergency medical care at sea are set down in many articles and in the preceding chapters of this book.

After you have done the fast first-aid maneuvers, i.e., restored breathing, stopped major bleeding, and gotten the victim out of further danger, questions arise. Is this a serious injury? What is likely to be the eventual outcome? Do I need help or can I manage? If I need help but can't get it in a hurry, what can I do for the patient?

FRACTURES

Fractures may be simple (i.e., no wound in continuity with the broken-bone ends), or compound, in which there is a wound in continuity with broken-bone ends. Each presents different prognosis and treatment.

It is obvious first off that, unless there is marked angulation of the part, you can't be sure there is a broken bone. However, if there is a severe sprain type of injury, it will do no harm to treat the injury as a fracture—provided you pay proper attention to the splinting.

Fractures of the fingers, wrist, forearm and arm, lower leg and ankle, when correctly aligned and splinted, can be cared for satisfactorily aboard for several days to a week. It is advisable to get help, but little harm will be done by an unavoidable delay of five or ten days. If there is to be a longer delay—two weeks or more—and if the shipboard reduction has been incomplete, a refracture may be needed later. This will prolong disability but does not exclude a satisfactory long-term result. Meanwhile, shipboard splinting makes the victim comfortable and minimizes further injury to soft tissue from the broken-bone ends.

Fractures about the elbow and extensive fractures at the ankle may interfere with the circulation of the arm or foot beyond the fracture site. Attention to general alignment and proper splinting are essential to avoid this.

Compound fractures (those with an open wound in continuity with the broken-bone ends) present an entirely different problem. Unless the open wound is properly cleaned, it permits infection of the bone ends (osteomyelitis) and this will greatly hinder healing. If there is to be a delay of more than 6 to 8 hours in evacuating a patient with a compound fracture, you can prevent osteomyelitis by washup of the wound, splinting of the extremity plus systemic antibiotic therapy. There is greater urgency in evacuating such a patient than one with a simple fracture. The wound must be dressed frequently to keep it clean and sweet-smelling.

A simple fracture of a long bone properly splinted, or a compound fracture washed up and splinted, requires many weeks to heal, and although medical care is desirable as expeditiously as possible, unavoidable delay of a couple of weeks need cause no serious anxiety.

Fractures of the clavicle and of the ribs will heal without exception. If enough ribs are broken to cause a flail chest (that is, there is enough interference with the rigidity of the chest wall so that the lung will not expand when a breath is taken) this threatens life. Place enough weight onto the fractured ribs (lead sinkers in a sock) to stabilize the chest wall.

BURNS

Burns are deceptive injuries. A large second-degree burn involving a chest and abdomen with blisters and redness, but preserving sensation to pinprick, is a painful and terrible-looking injury. However, if it is less than 20% of the body's surface and infection is prevented, it can be treated successfully aboard and will heal. It need occasion little alteration of cruise plans.

Burns of second or third degree involving more than 20% of the body's surface as determined by the Rule of Nines (see Fig. 22) may develop burn shock 8 to 24 hours after injury. If medical help can be gotten within that time, it should be. If not, heroic efforts must be made on board if the burn patient is to survive.

Third-degree burns of more than 10% of the body's surface, or an extremity, can be extremely serious, since such wounds result in a complete loss of skin and do not heal without a skin graft. Medical facilities are essential for this and evacuation within a period of days is desirable. However, if the wound is properly dressed, a delay of two or three weeks will not greatly increase the eventual disability.

Severe local third-degree burns, such as charring of an extremity (which is rare except with flame burns), often results in the dead tissue of the burned part forming a nidus for spreading infection. Unless evacuation is possible, systemic antibiotics and meticulous dressing of the wound can reduce the danger.

Sunburn rarely causes dangerous symptoms except in redheaded persons with a minimum of skin pigment. Even when blisters develop, unless severe infection ensues, recovery with no sequelae is the rule.

ABDOMINAL PAIN

Bellyache is a common complaint—usually not serious unless it persists. A surgical aphorism states that a previously healthy person who develops severe abdominal pain that lasts for more than 8 hours probably has surgical abdominal disease. The enema is a useful diagnostic aid, since constipation—particularly in the young—is a common cause of bellyache. Enema does no harm and may resolve the problem.

The most common surgical disease of the abdomen is acute appendicitis, particularly, though not exclusively, in the young. Cholecystitis or gallbladder infection is a middle-distance second. It most often strikes the overweight middle-aged individual. Perforated duodenal ulcer is a distant third. There are many other causes for abdominal surgical disease, but statistics indicate that you are most likely to encounter one of these three.

The history of appendectomy eliminates appendicitis. It sounds obvious, but don't forget to ask first off! Persons with gallbladder disease usually have had prior trouble that may range from mild indigestion and intolerance to rich food to a severe colic with previous major abdominal attacks.

Perforation is unlikely to be the initial symptom of a duodenal ulcer disease. A recent or remote history of treatment for ulcer by a physician will help. A history of pain around the umbilicus when the stomach is empty (hunger pains) that is relieved by food or antacid, points toward ulcer disease.

The pain of abdominal surgical disease usually starts distributed over the abdomen and in the course of hours localizes over the affected organ which then becomes tender when pressed upon. Tenderness in the right lower abdomen points to the appendix; in the right upper abdomen at the edge of the rib cage, to the gallbladder. Pain of appendicitis is often gradual in onset. That of a gallbladder disease may be gradual or severe depending upon whether or not a gallstone plugs the ductal system. If the latter happens, severe colic may start the attack.

Perforation of a duodenal ulcer presents a dramatic event—sudden overwhelming pain around the umbilicus, often a shock-like state, and the rapid development (in minutes to hours) of generalized tenderness and a rigidity of the entire abdomen called "board-like abdomen." The abdomen thumps exactly like a board.

You aren't likely to become a diagnostician from these few observations. However, you can decide with reasonable assurance whether you are dealing with a medical abdominal disease such as dysentery, "intestinal flu," dietary indiscretion, or a surgical condition. Fortunately, shipboard treatment for surgical abdominal disease (detailed elsewhere) is similar regardless of the cause. It also is essentially harmless should your diagnosis be incorrect. So, it is wiser to over- rather than undertreat.

A word of warning. Attempt no abdominal operation at sea. You may have read of heroic "appendectomies" performed by laymen or paramedics on ships at sea. These are all near-disasters. The victims survive in spite of, and not with the aid of, such ill-advised attempts. Surgical abdominal disease need not be fatal if immediate operation is not performed. If the body's defense mechanisms are supported, as you can do, the patient can arrive in port in salvageable condition.

One condition peculiar to women deserves special mention—mittleschmerz. Midway between two menstrual periods, the normal woman ovulates. An ovum ruptures the surface of the ovary and starts its descent toward the fallopian tube for possible fertilization. Such rupture usually passes unnoticed, but on occasion, may cause sudden right-lower or left-lower (if the left ovary is ovulating) abdominal pain. If there is a bit of blood spilled into the free abdominal cavity from the rupture, this may cause lower abdominal tenderness that simulates appendicitis. It differs though and of prime importance is timing. It occurs ten to fifteen days after the conclusion of the last menstrual period—hence its name, middle sickness or mittleschmerz. It is sudden in onset, as might be expected, and gets well spontaneously in a day or two. Tenderness is very low in the abdomen just above the pubic bone, and is accompanied by no upper abdominal distress such as is the case with appendicitis.

HEAT EXHAUSTION AND HEATSTROKE

Heat exhaustion is an acute condition due to excessive loss of salt and water from the body. Satisfactory replacement is possible without interruption of the cruise.

Heatstroke is an acute, dangerous condition. Treatment must be begun immediately, prompt recovery is sought, and protection from heat and sunlight for the remainder of the voyage is necessary for the victim of heatstroke.

DISLOCATIONS AND SPRAINS

Finger and toe dislocations can be reduced readily, particularly shortly after injury. Shoulder dislocations require drugs and more complex maneuvers, but reduction is possible.

Ankle sprains, properly taped, will support light duty. Any dislocation or sprain may have an accompanying fracture. If this is small, that is, without gross angulation, it will not be diagnosed without an X-ray examination. It never does harm to treat a severe sprain (massive swelling, severe pain and discoloration) as though a fracture is present. If recovery is complete within three to four weeks from a severe ankle sprain, it is unlikely that fracture was present.

WOUNDS

Soft-part wounds are of great variety. Those resulting from sharp instruments present clean cuts with regular margins. After hemostasis (stopping the bleeding), proper washup and closure of the skin, evacuation is not urgent unless major tendons or nerves have been cut. Inability to raise the fingers suggests transection of the extensor tendons at the wrist or hand. Inability to bend the fingers suggests a division of the flexor tendons at the wrist or hand. Numbness of the palm, thumb and first three fingers suggests a transection of the median nerve at the wrist.

Such nerve and tendon injuries are best repaired within two to three weeks of injury. Merely clean and close the wound over these structures. This gives the surgeon a healed wound to work through later on and is most desirable. As a matter of fact, many surgeons presently prefer to close the wound, allow it to heal, and do the repair of major nerve and tendon injuries after an interval of from two weeks to two months.

Jagged, irregular wounds of crush or tearing type, particularly if the skin is avulsed, should not be closed. After a good washup, pack them open. Evacuation of the patient is then desirable, because repeated dressings of such wounds is difficult and time-consuming. These patients also require systemic antibiotic treatment.

Any wound, clean, lacerated or rough-jagged, may become infected. Evacuation becomes pressing in this case since the problems of wound care and the possibility of systemic infection are present and require complicated treatment.

HEAD INJURY—THE UNCONSCIOUS PATIENT

Head injury accompanied by loss of consciousness is always of grave concern and a rough estimate of the extent of the brain damage is gained by the length of period of unconsciousness. After consciousness returns, complications may develop in the days following. Persistent and increasing headache, fainting or violent vomiting without nausea indicate force-10 weather ahead for the sufferer and urgent need for neurosurgical care.

Any crewman who is persistently unconscious from head injury, high fever or whatever cause, cannot be well cared for aboard a small vessel.

You must immediately supply fluids parenterally, keep the airway clear of mucus, provide for urinary drainage, and often, fecal incontinence. It is a major task in a hospital with all facilities. In my opinion, this situation urgently requires evacuation of the patient.

HEART ATTACK AND PENETRATING CHEST WOUNDS

These catastrophes require major hospital facilities as soon as possible. Certain fundamentals of care are available if evacuation of the patient is impossible. The patient with either of these conditions should be treated as a bunk patient until he can be moved to a medical facility.

Cardiac Arrest

If your efforts succeed in restoring heart action, the same rule applies as for patients with a heart attack.

SEVERE INFECTIONS

Serious bronchitis, pneumonia, throat and urinary tract infections are characterized by general malaise, often chills, high fever, plus symptoms pointing to the organ system involved. Cough, chest pain and shortness of breath indicate serious pulmonary disease—likely pneumonia. Red, sore throat with pain on swallowing often with enlarged lymph nodes in the neck indicates severe sore throat. Similar general symptoms together with frequency, urgency and burning on urination suggests bladder or kidney infection.

Such persistent illnesses with temperatures of from 102° F. to 103° F. by mouth for two days indicate an infection that merits trial of antibiotic therapy—this detailed elsewhere (*see* Chapters III, IV, VI—VIII) and may be successful before help arrives. Failure of response to antibiotics may indicate a virus infection that will not respond to antibiotic drugs.

VENEREAL DISEASE

Gonorrhea and syphilis are increasingly prevalent in our culture. These can be treated by proper antibiotic therapy aboard, but follow-up examination in six months is essential.

GLOSSARY

Limited definition of terms as used in medical practice.

Acid Chyme. Mixture of food, hydrochloric acid, pepsin and rennin enzymes fashioned in the stomach during digestion of food.

Anaphylaxis. Severe collapse that occurs when individual is challenged by a food or drug to which he is highly allergic. Can be fatal.

Antibacterial. Any substance harmful to bacteria.

Antibody. Immune substance produced in the living body when it is challenged by a foreign protein.

Antiemetic. Drugs or substances to stop or prevent vomiting.

Arm. Upper extremity from elbow to shoulder.

Asepsis. The technique of making a wound sterile by removing or destroying all bacteria.

Aspiration. Inhaling fluids or solids into the lungs. Occurs when patient is unconscious and gag and cough reflexes are depressed.

Bedsore. Weak or paralyzed patients may lie too long on one spot, squeeze the blood from it, the tissue dies and falls away, leaving an open sore.

Bilirubin. Bile pigment derived from hemoglobin breakdown.

Bilirubinuria. Excess bile in urine. Makes urine an orange color—accompanies jaundice.

Boardlike Abdomen. Rigid abdomen that feels as hard as a table. Accompanies perforated ulcer or other viscus.

Bowel Obstruction. Blockage of flow of bowels. May be mechanical (as with impaction) or reflex (as in peritonitis) from interruption of nerve impulses.

Bulb Syringe. Wide glass barrel with rubber bulb. Similar to a douche syringe or a turkey baster.

Butterflies. Adhesive tape bridges to close a wound.

Chemotherapeutic. Chemical agents (sulfa drugs and related compounds) that have antibacterial action.

Clitoris. Female analogy of male penis.

Coma. Loss of conscious response. Varies in degree and duration. Caused by blows, infections or severe imbalance of body chemistry, as diabetic coma.

Cubic Centimeter. Fluid volume measure. One one-thousandth of a liter.

Duodenum. First 12 inches of small intestine.

Enteric Coated. Outer coating for pill that will dissolve in small intestine rather than the stomach (i.e., salt pill).

Enzymes. Substances that are necessary for a chemical reaction but do not change character as a result of such reactions.

Fibroblasts. Young connective tissue cells that mature into scar.

Flaccid Paralysis. Completely limp paralysis, usually of an extremity. Often seen in head injury and stroke with unconsciousness.

Forearm. Upper extremity from elbow to wrist.

Genitourinary Tract. Urinary tract plus genitals. Male = penis and testes. Female = ovaries, fallopian tubes, uterus, clitoris, labia, and vagina.

Great Omentum. A fold of peritoneal (abdominal lining) membrane that swings free from lower edge of stomach. Known as "the abdominal policeman" because it is somewhat mobile and hastens to site of perforation or infection in abdominal organ and seals it off.

Groin. Crease between the lower abdomen and upper thigh.

Healing by First Intention. Primary healing of a wound without infection or delay.

Healing by Second Intention. Healing of a wound which has been infected and/or separated and must fill in with scar tissue.

Hematoma. A blood clot in the body tissues.

Homeostatic Mechanism. Those body organ systems that keep internal environment (temperature, acid/base balance, fluid volumes) quite constant despite varying demands from the environment.

Jaundice. Yellow color of skin and eyeballs due to retention of bile in the system.

Leg. Lower extremity from knee to ankle.

Leucocytes. White blood cells.

Lymph Node. Nodule of filtering tissue in the lymphatic fluid system.

Metabolism. The sum total of chemical activity in the living body.

Milliliter. One one-thousandth of a liter—liquid measure. *See* **Cubic Centimeter.**

Nasogastric Tube. A rubber or plastic tube for insertion through the nose, down the gullet and into the stomach. Suitably marked to indicate when it is in the stomach, it is used for emptying or filling the stomach.

Needle Holder. A toothed instrument to hold a curved needle for sewing tissue.

Neurons. Nerve cells.

Osteoblasts. Young connective tissue cells that mature into bony callus.

Outside Scrub. Washup and shaving of skin around a wound. Done before the wound washup.

Palpation. Examination by feeling with the hand.

Parenteral. Other than by mouth.

Penile. Relating to the male penis.

Perineum. Pelvic floor; underneath the crotch.

Phagocytosis. The ingestion of bacteria by white blood cells.

Pylorus. Circular sphincter muscle at the junction of the stomach and duodenum.

Rebound Tenderness. Tenderness experienced when firm hand pressure upon abdomen is suddenly released. Indicates peritoneal inflammation.

Serum. Liquid portion of blood exclusive of cells.

Spastic Paralysis. Paralysis of a limb but muscles are firmly contracted. Seen later on in head injury or stroke.

Subcutaneous. The region of fatty tissue immediately underneath the skin.

Suppository. Any drug so prepared as to be absorbed after insertion into the rectum.

Sutures. Surgical gobbledygook for stitches or thread.

Systemic. Antonym of local with regard to body processes, injury and disease.

Tenderness. Pain experienced when a part of the body is pressed upon.

Therapeutic Test. Use of treatment to help make a diagnosis.

Therapy. Treatment.

Thigh. Lower extremity from knee to groin.

Toothed Tissue Forceps. Tweezers with teeth for holding tissues.

Urinary Tract. Kidneys, ureters (tubes from kidneys to bladder), urinary bladder, urethra (tube from bladder to outside). Male has prostate gland and penis. Female has much shorter urethra.

Vasoconstriction. Narrowing or closing down of blood vessels.

Vasodilation. Dilation of blood vessels.

W.N.L. Within Normal Limits. Abbreviation used in describing results of physical examination.

Wound. Any solution of continuity of the architecture of a body tissue or tissues.

Wound Washout. Actual scrubbing and rinsing the depths of a wound. Also called wound toilet.

INDEX

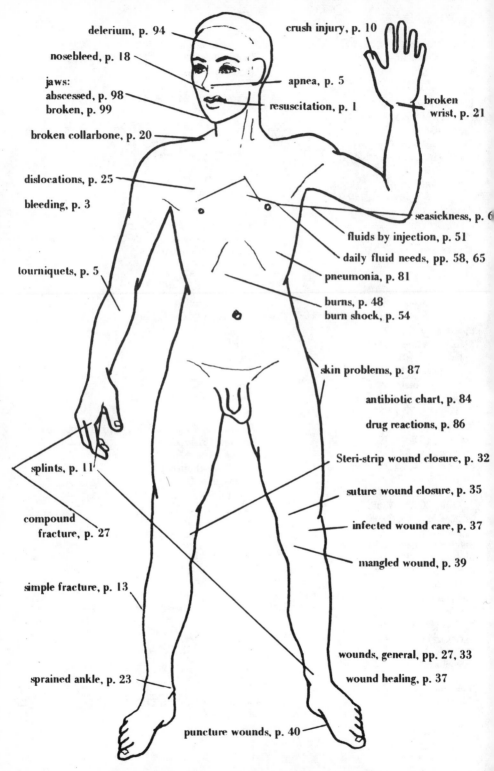

delerium, p. 94

crush injury, p. 10

nosebleed, p. 18

jaws:
abscessed, p. 98
broken, p. 99

broken collarbone, p. 20

apnea, p. 5

resuscitation, p. 1

broken
wrist, p. 21

dislocations, p. 25

bleeding, p. 3

seasickness, p. 6

fluids by injection, p. 51

daily fluid needs, pp. 58, 65

tourniquets, p. 5

pneumonia, p. 81

burns, p. 48
burn shock, p. 54

skin problems, p. 87

antibiotic chart, p. 84

drug reactions, p. 86

Steri-strip wound closure, p. 32

splints, p. 11

suture wound closure, p. 35

infected wound care, p. 37

compound
fracture, p. 27

mangled wound, p. 39

simple fracture, p. 13

wounds, general, pp. 27, 33

wound healing, p. 37

sprained ankle, p. 23

puncture wounds, p. 40

Rapid Reference to Recipes for Injury or Illness